CW00954321

Anaemia

A Guide to Causes, Treatment and Prevention

By the same author:

*Irritable Bowel Syndrome: Special Diet Cookbook
(with Ann Page-Wood)*

Premenstrual Syndrome: Special Diet Cookbook

The Essential Anaemia Cookbook

ANAEMIA

A Guide to Causes, Treatment and Prevention

Jill Davies

Thorsons

An Imprint of HarperCollins*Publishers*

Thorsons
An imprint of HarperCollins*Publishers*
77-85 Fulham Palace Road
Hammersmith, London W6 8JB

First published by Thorsons 1993
10 9 8 7 6 5 4 3 2 1

© Jill Davies 1993

Jill Davies asserts the moral right to be
identified as the author of this work

A catalogue record for this book
is available from the British Library

ISBN 0 7225 2846 9

Illustrations by Peter Cox

Typeset by Harper Phototypesetters Limited,
Northampton, England
Printed in Great Britain by
HarperCollinsManufacturing Glasgow

All rights reserved. No part of this publication may be
reproduced, stored in a retrieval system, or transmitted,
in any form or by any means, electronic, mechanical,
photocopying, recording or otherwise, without the prior
permission of the publishers.

Contents

Health Warning

Do not follow any of the advice given in this book without first checking with your medical practitioner that it is safe for you to do so.

Measurements

Metric

 g = gram
 mg = milligram or one-thousandth of a gram
 μg = microgram or one-millionth of a gram
 kg = kilogram or 1,000 grams
 ml = millilitre or one-thousandth of a litre
 l = litre or 1,000 millilitres

Imperial

 tsp = teaspoon or 5 millilitres
 tbs = tablespoon or 15 millilitres
 oz = ounce or 28.3 grams (30g)
 lb = pound or 16 ounces or 453 grams (455g)
 pt = pint or 20 fluid ounces or 570 millilitres (568ml)

American

 American standard cupful = 8 fluid ounces

Recommended Dietary Allowances*

Designed for the maintenance of good nutrition of practically all healthy people in the United States.

Age (years)	Iron (mg)	B_{12} (µg)	Folate (µg)
Males			
11-14	12	2.0	150
15-18	12	2.0	200
19-24	10	2.0	200
25-50	10	2.0	200
51 +	10	2.0	200
Females			
11-14	15	2.0	150
15-18	15	2.0	180
19-24	15	2.0	180
25-50	15	2.0	180
51 +	10	2.0	180
Pregnant	30	2.2	400
Lactating			
1st 6 months	15	2.6	280
2nd 6 months	15	2.6	260

* The allowances, expressed as average daily intakes over time, are intended to provide for individual variations among most normal persons as they live in the United States under usual environmental stresses.

Figures in the table come from Recommended Dietary Allowances 10th Edition Subcommittee on the Tenth Edition of the RDA's Food and Nutrition Board Commission on Life Sciences National Research Council National Academy Press Washington, D.C. 1989.

CHAPTER ONE

Introduction to Anaemia

Anaemia is considered to be a major health problem. According to the World Health Organization, about 30 per cent of people throughout the world suffer from anaemia. The most common cause is *iron deficiency*, and women have a higher incidence of *iron-deficiency anaemia* than men. Recent figures from hospitals in England and Wales have demonstrated that the ratio of women to men discharged from hospital for iron-deficiency anaemia was approximately 2:1.

Iron deficiency is not the only cause of anaemia. It can also stem from a lack of certain nutrients, such as vitamin B12; cancer therapy involving radiography or anti-cancer drugs or inherited defects such as sickle cell anaemia. However, as these 'other' types of anaemia are not as common as iron-deficiency anaemia and are not particularly considered as female problems, this book will focus on iron-deficiency anaemia.

Whatever the underlying cause for developing anaemia, the symptoms in general terms are very much the same. If you have anaemia you will be all too familiar with the following.

Symptoms check-list

- You are likely to suffer from headaches.
- You may feel tired and weak and the extent to which you experience this will depend upon whether your condition is mild or severe.
- The tiredness and weakness could make you become lethargic.

- Exertion, such as during exercise, may result in feelings of dizziness and you may feel that you are short of breath and experience palpitations (awareness of the heart beat, rapid heart action, abnormal rhythm and anxiety).

- You may develop pallor (paleness) in the creases in the skin, the lining of the mouth and inside the eyelids. Do note that it is misleading to diagnose anaemia by pallor alone.

- You may have other symptoms: for example, if you suffer from iron-deficiency anaemia your nails may be brittle.

To understand what iron-deficiency anaemia is, and how to cope with it, you need to know some important facts about iron.

Iron in the body

In ancient Eastern Mediterranean civilizations, iron was considered to be of heavenly origin. The so-called 'metal of heaven' was used for medicinal purposes in Egypt and Babylon. The amount of iron in the human body is small and is considered to be in the region of about 4g, yet despite this seemingly small quantity, iron is one of the most important elements essential for good health. All cells making up the human body contain iron.

By far the lion's share of iron in the body is found in blood, packaged inside the red blood cells. Here, it is in the form of *haemoglobin* (the oxygen-carrying protein of the red blood cells). About 80 per cent of the iron in the body is found inside the red blood cells as haemoglobin. The origin of the term haemoglobin is quite logical: *haem* means blood, *globin* is globular protein. The amount of haemoglobin present inside the red blood cells - which, by the way, are called *erythrocytes* - determines the actual colour of the red blood cells. Haemoglobin is therefore known as the blood pigment.

A fair amount of iron is found in the cells making up muscles in the body. The iron inside these muscle cells is in the form of *myoglobin* (the oxygen-holding protein of the muscle cells). We already know that globin refers to protein, and as I am sure you have deduced, *myo* means muscle. Myoglobin, like haemoglobin, is also a pigment and is responsible for the colour of muscles. To understand this, think about the colour of chicken flesh – typically, the breast is made up of light meat and the legs of dark meat. These differences in colour are a reflection of the amount of myoglobin present in the muscles. The leg meat is darker than the breast meat as the legs contain more myoglobin.

Iron is found in many *enzymes* (proteins which act as catalysts, and at very low concentrations increase the rate of chemical reactions). These enzymes are found inside the body cells and are known as intracellular iron-containing enzymes.

The role of iron

Energy is essential for life and in order for energy to be generated, iron is a vital ingredient. If we think about the roles of haemoglobin, myoglobin and the intracellular iron-containing enzymes the picture will become clearer:

● Haemoglobin picks up oxygen in the lungs and carries it by way of the blood system to all body tissues.

● Myoglobin holds oxygen in readiness for muscular activity and the iron is made available for muscle contraction.

● Intracellular iron-containing enzymes play an important role in respiration in the body cells.

Iron terminology is quite fascinating. The iron described so far has been associated with a particular role in the body. This iron is described as *functional iron*. However, the human body may have additional iron. Healthy people have a store of iron in their bodies which is described aptly as *storage iron*. This type of iron acts as a reserve; when the functional iron runs out it is replaced by storage iron.

Storage iron is found in the bone marrow (the soft material in the centre of long bones), liver (the largest gland in the body) and spleen (the largest endocrine/ductless gland in the body). In healthy adult men the iron store may amount to approximately 1g of iron, which is about one-quarter of the total body iron. However, in some people iron stores may be low or even non-existent for various reasons – for example, a woman with heavy monthly periods may have a diminished iron store. When the iron stores are depleted the individual is said to be in a state of *iron deficiency*.

Iron is stored as *ferritin* (an iron-protein complex) and *haemosiderin* (a conglomeration of ferritin). Special proteins are found in the cells lining the small intestine to enable the body to obtain iron from the diet. These cells are called *mucosal cells* and contain two particular proteins that help with the absorption of iron.

- Mucosal transferrin is the protein which transfers the iron to a carrier in the blood for transport called *blood transferrin*.
- *Mucosal ferritin* holds some iron in reserve in the mucosal cell. This is summarized in Figure 1.1.

If the body needs this reserve of iron inside the mucosal cells, the iron is released into the body. If the iron is not required, it is eventually lost as a result of wear and tear as food material passes through the gastrointestinal tract. The mucosal cells have a life span of about three days, after which time they are shed into the faeces. The iron stored in the mucosal cells provides a short-term buffer.

Once the iron is captured by the blood protein transferrin, it is carried to the bone marrow and other blood-manufacturing sites. All the body tissues take up the amount of iron that is needed. If there is any surplus iron the storage proteins in the bone marrow, liver and spleen take up the iron and store it.

RED BLOOD CELLS
If you think back to the fact that most of the iron in the body is found inside the red blood cells, it stands to reason that the bone marrow will take up large quantities of iron to enable red

Figure 1.1 *Absorption of iron in the gastrointestinal tract*

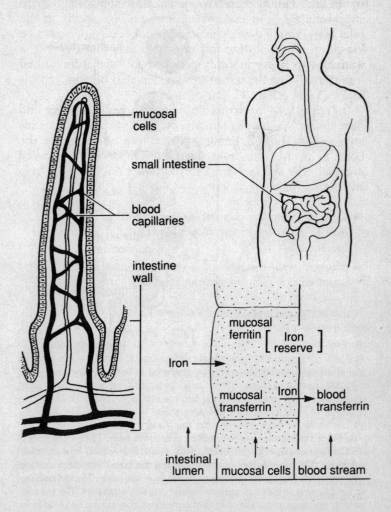

The absorption of iron takes place in the small intestine. Millions of tiny hair-like projections, called *villi*, increase the surface area of the small intestine so that iron and other nutrients are absorbed in a few hours. Inside the mucosal cells, iron may be held in reserve (by mucosal ferritin) or transferred by means of a carrier protein, mucosal transferrin, to a carrier protein in the blood, called blood transferrin.

Figure 1.2   *Red blood cell formation* (Haemopoiosis)

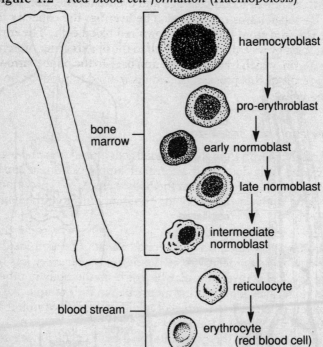

Red blood cells, the erythrocytes, are produced in bone marrow from stem cells, the haemocytoblasts. These cells divide to form erythroblasts (pro-erythroblast, early, intermediate and late normoblasts). During this time the cells change their appearance and accumulate haemoglobin. The red cells released from the bone marrow enter the blood stream as reticulocytes.

Red blood cells are among the smallest cells in the body. These cells are the most numerous type in the blood, with about five million to one cubic millimetre. The red cells are biconcave discs and this gives them a large surface area which lets them take up oxygen efficiently in the lungs. The red cells are soft and flexible so they can squeeze through the tiny capillaries. The red cells are not very tough and as they don't have a nucleus, they cannot divide to form new cells. Thousands of new red cells are needed every second to replace the ones that die.

blood cells to be made. Figure 1.2 shows the sequence of events involved in the production of red blood cells.

Red blood cells circulate in the blood for approximately four months, then are destroyed in the liver and spleen. Despite the fact that the red blood cells age and eventually die, iron from the haemoglobin is not wasted. The liver has the capacity to save the iron from the broken-down red blood cells. The iron is recycled by way of attaching itself to the blood carrier protein transferrin, which transports the iron back to the bone marrow. As a result of this process, the iron is re-used to produce new blood cells.

How the body loses iron

Although the iron from the red blood cells is used over and over again, the body does need a constant supply of iron, as small amounts of iron are lost from the body daily. As we know from scientific study, our capacity for excreting iron from the body is limited.

Approximately 1 mg of iron is lost daily by way of the gastrointestinal tract, urine, skin and sweat. The iron lost in this way may be referred to as the *minimal obligatory loss* or *basal loss*. Of course, iron may be lost from the body in other ways such as bleeding, during menstruation for example (page 22). Nevertheless, irrespective of additional losses of iron it is essential that these basal losses are replaced.

Iron losses from the gastrointestinal tract occur for several reasons. The cells lining the tract – the mucosal cells – are lost as a consequence of a process called *desquamation*. The amount of iron lost in this way is about 0.14 mg. A tiny amount of blood is lost too, which means that the iron in the haemoglobin is wasted. This is usually of the order of 0.38 mg. Bile which is produced in the liver contains iron and this leaves the body by way of the gastrointestinal tract. Daily losses of iron in bile are about 0.24 mg.

The amount of iron lost in urine is about 0.1 mg per day. This is likely to come from desquamated cells of the urinary tract together with small quantities of red blood cells.

Losses of iron from the skin are described as *dermal losses*. Contrary to popular belief, the iron losses from this source are negligible. Some of the early studies on iron balance suggested that people living in hot climates, those engaged in heavy physical work or athletes involved in endurance sports might be at risk for iron losses as a result of sweating. A recent study reported in The American Journal of Clinical Nutrition concluded as follows: 'The basal iron requirements can thus be considered to be the same for subjects living in a temperate climate and subjects living in a hot climate as well as in subjects with marked sweat losses due to heavy physical work or engagement in endurance sports.'

Iron in the diet

Iron in the diet is obtained from a variety of food sources. It is interesting to look at diets in different countries as the major food contributors of dietary iron are dependent upon the food supply. In Morocco and Libya, for example, a significant proportion of iron is derived from fruit and vegetables. In Cameroon, more than 20 per cent of the iron comes from alcoholic beverages and tree crops. In some of the African countries a large proportion of the dietary iron is provided by staple foods such as millet, sorghum or maize.

In the United Kingdom, the Ministry of Agriculture, Fisheries and Food (MAFF) publishes an annual report, 'Household Food Consumption and Expenditure', produced by the National Food Survey Committee. Food records are obtained from a random sample of private households throughout the UK.

Recent figures from the National Food Survey indicate that the iron content of food obtained for consumption at home is about 10.6mg per day. Table 1.1 (see page 9) shows where this iron actually comes from: cereal foods come top, and collectively vegetables and fruit rank second in the iron league table. It is interesting to see that approximately two-thirds of the iron in the UK diet comes from plant sources, although meat and meat products are also important sources of iron.

The contribution of iron to the diet from cereals is worth looking into further. Breakfast cereals can provide a significant amount – on average 1.4mg of iron per person per day. This is in part due to the iron content of the cereal itself and in certain cases a result of fortification. Next time you visit the supermarket, do a quick scan of the cereal packets and note which ones are fortified. White bread and products made from

Table 1.1 Food sources of iron in the UK diet based on national averages*

Food	Iron mg/person per day
Cereals	5.0
Meat and meat products	1.9
Vegetables	1.8
Eggs	0.3
Fruit	0.3
Milk and milk products	0.3
Fish	0.2
Fats	0.1
Sugar	0.1
Other	0.6

* Figures from 'Household food consumption and expenditure 1989', Annual Report of the National Food Survey Committee by the Ministry of Agriculture, Fisheries and Food (HMSO, 1990).

white flour such as cakes, biscuits and pastries account for average daily intakes of 0.9 and 0.6 mg of iron respectively, as in the UK white flour is enriched with iron.

It probably comes as no surprise that meat is a useful source of iron. Within the meat group comes offal and despite the fact that this is generally thought of as being a rich source of iron, the amount eaten is so small that it only provides an average daily intake of 0.2mg of iron per person.

The National Food Survey gives a general idea about food consumption in the home, and is therefore limited. The *Dietary and Nutritional Survey of British Adults* adds to the general picture. The aim of the survey was to recruit a nationally representative sample of adults aged between 16 and 64 living in private households in the UK and involved participants in keeping records of their total dietary intake for seven days. In terms of the total amount of iron in the diet, men took 14.0mg daily, women 12.3mg. Table 1.2 shows the average daily intakes of iron from main food groups.

A number of smaller studies have been carried out on

Table 1.2 Average daily intake of iron*

Food type	Iron mg/person per day
Cereal products	5.07
Meat and meat products	2.76
Vegetables	1.81
Beverages	0.51
Eggs and egg dishes	0.44
Fish and fish dishes	0.30
Fruit and nuts	0.30
Sugar, confectionery and preserves	0.24
Milk and products	0.22
Fats and spreads	0.04
Miscellaneous	0.41

* Figures from J. Gregory, K. Foster, H. Tyler and M. Wiseman, 'The dietary and nutritional survey of British adults', (HMSO, 1990).

vegetarians and strict vegetarians (vegans). Vegans live on a diet made up of plant foods only, yet it appears that intakes of iron do not go down as a consequence; in fact, an upward trend in iron intake has been demonstrated in a number of studies, particularly among vegans. This is encouraging for the many recent converts to vegetarian and vegan diets.

The absorption of iron

We now know that the average daily intake of iron is of the order of about 12 to 14 mg and that it comes from a wide variety of foods. We also know that special proteins in the lining cells of the small intestine play a vital role in the absorption of iron. However, the story does not end here.

According to the Food and Agriculture Organization of the United Nations, a diet typical for most segments of the population in industrialized countries comprises generous amounts of meat, poultry, fish and/or foods containing high amounts of vitamin C. Such a diet is considered to be of 'high bio-availability' with iron absorption of about 15 per cent. However the more recent panel on Dietary Reference Values in the UK, produced by the Department of Health, cautioned that iron in diets containing little or no meat is less well absorbed.

The iron taken in the diet that is not absorbed simply passes out of the body in the faeces when the bowels are opened. A 15 per cent absorption rate or even less appears to be rather wasteful. Why is the amount of iron absorbed considerably less than the amount taken in? To answer this question, it is necessary to know about different types of iron occurring in foods and factors that influence the absorption of dietary iron.

Most of the iron in the diet is called *non-haem iron*. This comprises all the iron found in foods of plant origin and some of the iron from foods of animal origin. The remaining iron is known as *haem iron*, which is only found in animal products. Haem iron is found in haemoglobin and myoglobin, and so it is not a surprise to find that it is present in foods such as meat, poultry and fish. Haem iron is highly available to the body as it is well absorbed. Non-haem iron is also found in the same foods as those containing haem iron. However, foods such as cereals, pulses, nuts, vegetables, fruit and dairy products only contain non-haem iron. This type of iron is not always easily absorbed by the body and is due to several factors:

- The chemical state of the iron.
- Substances hindering absorption.
- The iron status of the individual.

For absorption to take place, the non-haem iron needs to undergo a chemical change. This form of iron is described as *ferric* iron and in order for it to be absorbed it needs to be converted to *ferrous* iron. A number of substances have the ability to facilitate the change of state from ferric to ferrous (see Figure 1.3): *hydrochloric acid*, which is produced in the lining of the stomach and finds its way into gastric juice; *ascorbic acid*, commonly described as vitamin C in fruit and vegetables and *amino acids*, found in meat.

Non-haem iron is readily precipitated by a number of

substances that occur in foods and this may lead to poor absorption. Table 1.3 gives some examples. Perhaps we should then start thinking about the diet as a whole, instead of nutritional components existing in isolation.

Figure 1.3 *Factors involved in the conversion of ferric iron to ferrous iron**

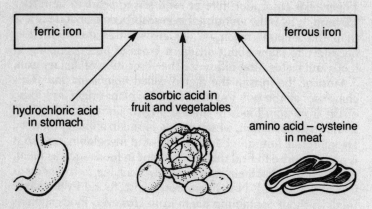

The iron status of an individual has a strong bearing on the absorption of non-haem iron and to a lesser extent on haem iron. As the amount of storage iron increases, the intestinal rate of absorption decreases. Similarly, if the body stores of iron decrease, there is an increase in the amount of iron absorbed.

If you are a logical person you are probably asking, 'If most of the iron in the diet is non-haem and the absorption of this is related to body stores, what's all the fuss about? Why do people develop iron deficiency anaemia at all?' To answer this question, we need to delve deeper and find out what iron-deficiency anaemia is all about.

Table 1.3 Some dietary factors involved in the precipitation of iron*

Precipitating agent	Food source	Insoluble complex formed
Oxalate	spinach	iron oxalate
Phosphate	rhubarb, egg yolk	iron phosphate
Phytate	wholegrain cereals and pulses	iron phytate
Tannin	tea, pulses, condiments and spices	iron tannate

CHAPTER TWO
What is Iron-Deficiency Anaemia?

Anaemia is a condition in which the oxygen carrying capacity of the blood is reduced. This occurs when the levels of oxygen carrying pigment or haemoglobin fall below normal. If you are in good health, the amount of haemoglobin circulating in your blood is stable and maintained by a strict balance. If the balance is upset, anaemia may result.

The symptoms of anaemia relate to the reduced oxygen carrying capacity of the blood. The severity of the symptoms depends on how low haemoglobin levels are. In women, normal blood haemoglobin concentrations range between 11.5g to 16g per 100mls of blood. If your haemoglobin level falls below 10g per 100ml of blood, you are likely to suffer from headaches and feel tired and lethargic. With a further reduction in haemoglobin levels to below 8g haemoglobin per 100ml of blood, you are likely to experience difficulty in breathing during exercise. You may feel dizzy because of the lack of oxygen getting to the brain. The reduced supply of oxygen may have an effect on the muscles of the heart, resulting in palpitations. This happens because the heart muscle has to work harder to compensate for the lack of oxygen. The pallor that some people experience may be related to reduced amounts of haemoglobin in the blood; after all, haemoglobin is the red pigment found inside the red blood cells.

Iron-deficiency anaemia may be associated with other symptoms typical of iron deficiency states. The additional symptoms may include:

- Brittle nails
- Spoon-shaped nails, as opposed to concave nails
- Soreness of the tongue and corners of the mouth
- Swallowing difficulties

Another factor influencing the symptoms is the underlying cause of the condition. For example, if blood loss arising from a peptic ulcer is the cause of your anaemia, your symptoms may well include abdominal pain and black faeces.

What causes iron-deficiency anaemia?

Iron-deficiency anaemia develops if insufficient iron is available to the bone marrow where haemoglobin is made and packaged into the red blood cells. The red blood cell formation becomes defective. There are three main reasons why there may not be enough iron available for the production of haemoglobin:

- Blood loss, causing loss of iron from the body
- Poor absorption of iron from the diet
- Lack of iron in the diet

The main cause of iron-deficiency is loss of iron as a consequence of losing blood. Blood losses of iron may occur for a number of reasons. If you have particularly heavy periods, you may be vulnerable to iron deficiency anaemia. Certain diseases, particularly those of the digestive tract may be responsible for persistent bleeding, for example stomach cancer and haemorrhoids (the latter commonly referred to as piles). Prolonged treatment with aspirin and aspirin-like nonsteroidal anti-inflammatory drugs may cause gastro-intestinal bleeding. In some parts of the world, hookworm infestation of the gastrointestinal tract is an important cause of iron-deficiency anaemia. You may not be aware of blood loss from the digestive tract - if it comes from the stomach or upper intestine it is invisible unless the loss is excessive, in which case the stools will be black in colour. If the loss of blood is lower down the digestive tract, it is more likely to be noticed in the faeces as it is bright red in colour. Diseases of the urinary tract such as tumours of the kidneys and bladder and cystitis (inflammation of the bladder) can cause blood loss, which tends to colour the urine.

The second most common cause of iron deficiency is poor absorption of iron from the diet. This may be as a result of surgical removal of part or all of the stomach. Coeliac disease, also known as gluten enteropathy, is a condition in which the lining of the small intestine is damaged by gluten (a protein derived from wheat and other cereals), causing malabsorption. Failure to absorb nutrients from the small intestine can lead to mineral deficiencies and anaemia.

The third possible cause of iron deficiency is a diet that does not provide enough iron. Lack of iron in the diet is more particularly associated with old people who live alone and who eat a poor diet. Children and pregnant women may not have enough iron in their diets to meet the additional demands for iron associated with growth and the specific needs of pregnancy. People on slimming diets may have low intakes of iron as a direct result of low food intake.

DIAGNOSIS OF IRON-DEFICIENCY ANAEMIA
If you think you have iron-deficiency anaemia, seek the advice of your medical practitioner. DO NOT SELF-DIAGNOSE. You can help your doctor by giving an accurate account of any symptoms you have experienced. You could take along any medication that you are on that the doctor does not know about, such as aspirin, as we know that prolonged use of this can cause gastrointestinal bleeding. If you have piles, don't conceal this, as loss of blood arising from this disorder will be highly relevant to the diagnosis. Likewise, if your periods are heavy, do not withhold this information. If you have been attempting to slim, this should be mentioned because low energy intake tends to mean low iron intake. Put your doctor fully in the picture.

Medical diagnosis can be made from taking a sample of your blood and carrying out specific tests:

● *Measurement of haemoglobin* whereby anaemia is usually

defined as a concentration of haemoglobin below a particular arbitrary value. If your haemoglobin concentration is below 120g per litre of blood or 110g if you are pregnant, you will be diagnosed as anaemic. In men the threshold level is higher at 130g per litre of blood.

● *Examination of a blood film* whereby a sample of blood is looked at under a microscope. If you have severe iron deficiency anaemia your red blood cells will be smaller and paler than normal (Figure 2.1). In medical terms, the small cells are described as *microcytic* and the reduction in colour of the cells makes them *hypochromic*. This type of anaemia is therefore referred to as microcytic and hypochromic anaemia.

● *Other tests* may be carried out in connection with the diagnosis if your doctor is unclear about the underlying cause of your anaemia. You may be asked to provide a specimen of faeces for analysis for evidence of blood. You may need to have more invasive tests such as a barium X-ray examination or endoscopy to find out if you have a disorder of the gastrointestinal tract.

Figure 2.1 *Red blood cells in a healthy person and in iron-deficiency anaemia*

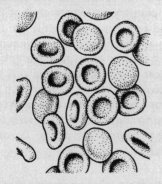 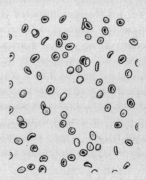

● Red blood cells about 7 micrometres in diameter
● red in colour
● full complement of haemoglobin

● red blood cells smaller
● paler in colour
● reduced haemoglobin level

Not just iron-deficiency anaemia

The Department of Health makes it very clear that iron deficiency can have an effect on the following:

- Work capacity
- Intellectual performance
- Behaviour
- Resistance to infection
- Body temperature

WORK CAPACITY

A number of very interesting studies have shown a relationship between haemoglobin levels and work capacity. It was shown in some early studies that animals put on an iron-deficient diet near the time of weaning and made anaemic by bleeding or the administration of a particular drug became exhausted more quickly than when haemoglobin levels were 'normal'. Studies on humans have also shown that a relationship exists between haemoglobin levels and work capacity. Female tea estate workers in Sri Lanka with low haemoglobin levels were found to have reduced work capacity (determined by a treadmill test) than tea workers with higher blood concentrations of haemoglobin: this could have a marked effect on the economy of the country, as 50 per cent of the female tea workers were found to be iron-deficient. On the Pacific coast of Guatamala, it was found that anaemic plantation workers on a mixed coffee and sugar plantation performed less well in a step test than non-anaemic workers. Interestingly, the anaemic individuals were considered to be poor workers, lazy and stupid by the plantation owner. When iron supplementation was given to these workers the step test performance improved and they were observed to become more willing, intelligent and effective workers.

INTELLECTUAL PERFORMANCE

Studies on iron-deficiency anaemia and educational achievement are a bit thin on the ground, although a recent study in an economically deprived rural area of central Java,

Indonesia showed that iron supplementation among iron-deficient anaemic children benefits learning processes as measured by school achievement test scores. Clearly, much more work needs to be done on evaluating achievement in formal educational settings. It has been suggested that iron deficiency may have significant implications in terms of learning and ultimate scholastic performance.

BEHAVIOUR

It is well recognized that adults with iron-deficiency anaemia have a tendency towards apathy. Pediatricians have often described iron-deficient children as being irritable and uninterested in their surroundings, and studies on animals have given backing to these observations. Mice were reared to have a low level of iron in their brains. The young animals were then observed in a controlled environment and their behaviour for three minutes was monitored and compared with mice that were not iron-deficient. The iron-deficient mice were similar to the non-iron-deficient mice when walking and defecating, but there was a marked reduction in rearing on their hind legs and standing still. A study on infants in Guatamala based on assessing behavioural differences between anaemic and non-anaemic infants showed that anaemic infants differed markedly in terms of behavioural pattern (Table 2.1).

RESISTANCE TO INFECTION

The effect of iron deficiency on resistance to infection is very interesting. Early studies on animals in the 1930s showed that dogs and cats had increased parasitic infestation with iron deficiency. The earliest clinical report in 1928 showed that infants from poor families in London had a modest decrease in bronchitis and gastroenteritis when they received iron supplementation. More recently, iron deficiency with or without anaemia has been reported to increase chronic candidiasis (thrush) and recurrent herpes infection. The mechanisms that reduce resistance to infection with iron deficiency are uncertain and have only recently begun to be investigated.

Table 2.1   Differences between anaemic and non-anaemic infants*

Behaviour pattern	Number of infants	
	Anaemic	Non-anaemic
Withdrawn or hesitant	6	2
Fearful	7	2
Tense	7	1
Unreactive to usual stimuli	7	3
Decreased bodily activity	7	4
Lack of persistence	8	5

* Cited in N. S. Scrimshaw, 'Functional consequences of iron deficiency in human populations', *Journal of Nutrition Science and Vitaminology*, 30 (1984), 47-63.

BODY TEMPERATURE

Abnormalities in body temperature due to iron deficiency were first described in experimental animals. When compared to non-iron-deficient rats, iron-deficient rats that had been exposed to a temperature of 4°C for 6 hours showed a greater decrease in body temperature. A study carried out in Caracas, Venezuela with humans relaxing in a water bath which started at a temperature of 36°C and was rapidly lowered to 28°C for 1 hour resulted in those suffering with severe iron deficiency unable to maintain body temperature. 'Normal' subjects had a fall in oral temperatures of 0.2°C; iron-deficient subjects a fall of 0.5°C and iron-deficiency anaemic subjects a fall in oral temperature of 0.9°C. Much more needs to be known about iron deficiency and temperature regulation, but it is tempting to speculate about the importance of this, particularly in the case of old people living alone. Hypothermia in such people is often related to the high cost of fuel: perhaps iron-deficiency anaemia may exacerbate the condition.

CHAPTER THREE

Why Women are Vulnerable to Iron-Deficiency Anaemia

Women are more likely to develop iron-deficiency anaemia than men. Some of the reasons for this are quite obvious: for example, blood loss as a consequence of menstruation. But there are other reasons why women are particularly vulnerable.

Less body iron

Women have less iron in their bodies than men. In an adult man there are about 50mg of iron per kilogram of body weight, whereas in women there are approximately 35mg of iron per kilogram. In terms of amounts of iron in the body a man has about 3.5g of iron and a woman about 2.3g.

These figures are reflected in the amount of iron stored. The storage reserve of iron in men is about 1,000mg. In contrast the storage iron in women is much less, amounting to approximately 200 to 400mg.

If we now turn to the iron described as functional iron and examine normal blood haemoglobin concentrations it becomes apparent that haemoglobin levels in men are higher than they are in women. Haemoglobin concentrations in men are normally from 13.5g to 18g per 100 ml of blood, whereas in women, the normal blood concentrations are from 11.5g to 16g per 100 ml.

Lower intakes of iron

Women have lower intakes of iron than men (12.3mg per day and 14.0mg per day respectively) and this is associated with the fact that women have lower energy intakes than males. The differences in the amount of iron in the diets of the two sexes is probably to some extent a reflection of the tendency of women towards slimming diets. This trend is substantiated by the findings of a Dietary and Nutritional Survey of British adults. At the time the dietary records were completed, 12 per cent of the women and 4 per cent of the men reported that they were on slimming diets.

The need or the desire to slim does not necessarily mean that the diet has to lack iron. Sensible meal planning and the consumption of foods known to provide significant amounts of iron can immediately eradicate this potential problem.

Menstruation

Apart from the basal losses of iron as described on page 7 which amount to about 0.86mg per day, women have additional losses during the reproductive phase of their life cycle. The loss of blood on a monthly basis inevitably has implications for iron status. Menstrual blood loss is fairly constant from month to month – studies have shown that most women lose about 44ml of blood per cycle. This leads to an iron loss of about 19.8mg, which on a 28-day cycle averages 0.7mg per day.

While menstrual blood loss is fairly constant in the same individual, it varies widely between women. Having regard to iron losses through menstruation, the Food and Agriculture Organization have stated that 25 per cent of women lose more than 0.8mg of iron per day; 10 per cent more than 1.3mg per day; and 5 per cent more than 1.6mg per day on top of the basal loss of 0.86mg per day.

Clearly, heavy or prolonged periods need to be brought to the attention of medical experts and it may be necessary for iron supplements to be prescribed.

Pregnancy

The 'iron costs' of pregnancy are relatively high. Pregnant women require iron to replace basal losses and additional iron to meet the specific demands of pregnancy. During pregnancy additional iron is needed for a variety of reasons which include:

● Production of red blood cells
● Growth and development of the fetus
● Growth and development of the placenta
● Loss of blood when the baby is born

If the pregnant woman is enjoying good health and is well nourished, there is an average increase in haemoglobin iron by about 500mg during the pregnancy. When the baby is born its body contains approximately 290mg of iron and the placenta contains about 25mg of iron. As well as this, blood loss at delivery will result in further iron loss. The average blood loss when the baby is born has been estimated to be around 150mg, ranging from 90 to 310mg.

According to the Department of Health, all women of child bearing age should ideally have sufficient stores of iron to cope with the metabolic demands made by pregnancy. These demands should be met due to the cessation of menstrual losses, the mobilization of maternal iron stores and the increased intestinal absorption of iron. But the DOH makes one proviso: when iron stores are inappropriately low at the start of pregnancy, supplementation with iron may be necessary.

Clearly, if you are planning a pregnancy or if you think or know you are pregnant it is sensible to discuss any concerns about iron with your medical practitioner.

Breast feeding

There is a large volume of literature singing the praises of breast feeding with benefits to the health and well-being of both the mother and baby. For example, the mother will rid her body of fat laid down in pregnancy as a consequence of milk production, and the infant will be provided with anti-infective factors which are not found in artificial feeds.

On the iron front, breast milk is particularly advantageous to the infant because the iron in breast milk is very well absorbed. The bio-availability of this type of iron is approximately 50 per cent compared to about 10 to 20 per cent for cow's milk formula.

Breast feeding is associated with a saving in iron as a result of the absence of menstrual losses. After a baby is born several months elapse before menstruation recommences if the mother is breast feeding. The amount of iron that is secreted in breast milk roughly equals the saving from not having periods.

Intra-uterine devices

Women who practise birth control may be at risk of increased blood loss as a result of the method they choose to use. Methods of contraception have been found to have a marked influence on menstrual blood loss. Intra-uterine devices may double the rate of blood loss that occurs during menstruation. On the other hand, the use of oral contraceptives reduces menstrual blood loss by about half.

Clearly, the advice of a medical practitioner needs to be taken on this, taking account of individual medical histories. Not everyone is suited to the Pill, so it is not a straightforward switch from intra-uterine to oral contraception.

Donating blood

Obviously, giving blood results in a reduction in body iron. However, the moral in this story is not to stop giving blood (unless specifically advised to do so by a medical practitioner), but rather to pay careful attention to the length of time between the blood donations.

According to the National Blood Transfusion Service, regular blood donors who give blood at intervals of not less than 6 months are able to replenish their own iron stores. The Department of Health have suggested that this is probably achieved by means of an increased efficiency of absorption of iron. However, the DOH cautioned that more frequent donations, particularly by women of child-bearing age may warrant a higher intake of iron to maintain adequate iron status.

CHAPTER FOUR

How Much Iron to Aim For

What are dietary reference values?

The most recently published figures for nutrient intakes in the UK are found in the Department of Health report, 'Dietary Reference Values for Food Energy and Nutrients for the United Kingdom'. Table 4.1 gives a breakdown of the latest figures for iron intakes.

Undoubtedly, the figures need to be explained. The *Estimated Average Requirement* (EAR) gives a notional mean requirement of a group of people. About half will usually need more than the EAR and half, less. *The Reference Nutrient Intake* (RNI) is higher than the EAR and intakes above the RNI will be adequate for the majority of people. The *Lower Reference Nutrient Intake* (LNRI) represents the lowest intake which will meet the needs of some people, but intakes below this level are likely to be inadequate for most people.

Is your diet of high-bioavailability?

The type of foods you consume will be important. Assuming you are on a mixed diet containing generous quantities of meat, poultry, fish and/or foods containing high amounts of vitamin C you are likely to absorb about *15 per cent* of the iron in your diet. If your food choices are in the direction of a vegetarian diet and contain lots of vitamin C, the percentage absorbed is likely to be of the same order. However, poorly constructed vegetable based diets, low in vitamin C may result in a reduced absorption of iron, possibly around 10 per cent.

Table 4.1 Dietary Reference Values for iron expressed as milligrams iron per day*

Age (years)	Lower Reference Nutrient Intake	Estimated Average Requirement	Reference Nutrient Intake
11-18			
(males)	6.1	8.7	11.3
(females)	8.0	11.4	14.8
19-50			
(males)	4.7	6.7	8.7
(females)	8.0	11.4	14.8
50+			
(males/females)	4.7	6.7	8.7

The figures show that during their reproductive years women have additional requirements for iron compared with males and post-menopausal women. Girls or women with high menstrual losses may need to take iron supplements to increase iron intakes.

* Figures in the table come from 'Dietary Reference Values for Food Energy and Nutrients for the United Kingdom', Report of the Panel on Dietary Reference Values of the Committee on Medical Aspects of Food Policy, Department of Health (HMSO, 1991).

Therefore you need to be honest with yourself about the 'quality' of your diet.

How much iron needs to be replaced?

You should have some idea about the amount of iron you need to have in your daily diet. We have already established the fact that the body conserves iron very well and that basal losses are around 0.86 milligrams per day. The basal losses need to be replaced, so for starters you need 0.86mg of iron per day.

You need to try to estimate whether or not your periods are heavy. This is difficult to do and is a problem that has certainly vexed researchers on the subject of menstrual losses. Interestingly, in one study 40 per cent of women with a blood loss of about 80ml for one period considered their menstruation to be moderate or normal. Average losses in women are about 44ml, as previously discussed. This means a loss of 19.8mg of iron, which on a 28-day cycle averages 0.7mg per day. Heavy periods have yet to be defined, but the Department of Health states that a menstrual loss of 118ml per period will result in a loss of 1.90mg of iron per day over a 28-day cycle. As in the case of basal iron losses, menstrual iron losses need to be replaced.

Your iron needs

You will need to focus on the following:

- The percentage of iron likely to be absorbed from your diet; usually 15 per cent but possibly less.
- A basal loss of 0.86 milligrams iron per day.
- A menstrual loss equal to 0.7 milligrams iron per day or more.

Table 4.2   The amount of iron (expressed as mg per day) derived from Dietary Reference Values in relation to iron absorption

Absorption for iron (%)	Lower Reference Nutrient Intake (8.0mg)	Estimated Average Requirement (11.4mg)	Reference Nutrient Intake (14.8mg)
10	0.8	1.14	1.48
15	1.2	1.71	2.22

The figures show that the percentage of iron absorbed has an effect on the amount of iron taken into the body. The message is to go for a 'healthy' mixed diet.

Table 4.2 shows how much iron you would obtain from the

Dietary Reference Values assuming 10 and 15 per cent absorption of iron intake.

With these figures in mind, you now need to add your basal losses to your menstrual losses. If your periods are 'normal' you should need a total of 1.56mg of iron a day (0.86 + 0.7mg iron). On the other hand if your periods are heavy you could need as much as 2.76mg of iron per day (0.86 + 1.90mg iron).

In order to obtain 1.56mg of iron a day, you could achieve this from the EAR assuming a 15 per cent iron absorption. If your estimated absorption for iron is less (possibly as low as 10 per cent), you need to consider eating more foods of animal origin or lots of fresh fruit and vegetables. Alternatively, you could seek the advice of your doctor or health care professional regarding iron supplements.

An achievement of 2.76mg of iron per day is not in line with any of the figures in Table 4.2, although the nearest figure is provided by the RNI, assuming a 15 per cent absorption for iron. The DOH acknowledges that some women may need to take iron supplements when periods are heavy. In these circumstances, seek medical advice.

You may need more iron!

You may need to consider the need for more iron according to particular situations:

- If you are pregnant and have been on a poor diet. In such circumstances, your iron stores might be low.
- Your state of health may have to be considered. If you have piles, for example, you will have additional losses of body iron; similarly, if you have had an injury resulting in significant loss of blood.
- If you donate blood regularly you may possibly need to consider your dietary intake of iron.
- Keen sportswomen who are marathon runners may lose blood through stress. This usually comes out in urine and faeces.

It may be that the RNI will suffice, but all of these

circumstances merit discussion with your doctor. Iron supplements may well be prescribed.

CHAPTER FIVE

The Medicinal Approach

If you have been diagnosed by your doctor as having iron-deficiency anaemia or if you have been identified as a likely victim for developing the disorder, iron preparations may be prescribed. Essentially, your doctor is concerned with treatment (the course of action adopted to deal with the condition) and prophylaxis (the art of preventing the disorder from occurring). This is an important issue because iron preparations should only be prescribed for treatment and prophylaxis.

Assist your doctor

The type of preparation prescribed will depend upon your medical history. Help your doctor to help you by making a check-list:

● Are you already taking any self-medication? If so, tell your doctor because various drugs may interact with each other.

● Have you ever suffered with side-effects from iron preparations taken previously? If so, be sure to let your doctor know the details.

● Are you likely to be pregnant? If you think that this is possible let your doctor know.

Most iron preparations are designed to be taken by mouth and hence the term *oral iron*. However, in some circumstances it

Figure 5.1   *Oral administration of iron*

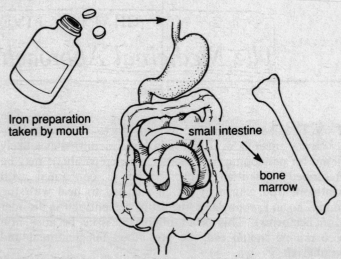

Iron preparation taken by mouth

small intestine

bone marrow

Orally administered iron is transported across the intestinal mucosa and is carried by transferrin to the bone marrow.

may be necessary to administer iron into a muscle or vein, and if this is the case the term *parenteral iron* is used. Figures 5.1 and 5.2 show the underlying principles of both oral and parental iron therapy respectively.

Iron by mouth

Pharmacological preparations containing iron and that can be swallowed come in four varieties:

1 *Tablets:* iron salts mixed with other ingredients, eg binding agents, compressed into a solid form, usually round in shape.
2 *Capsules:* iron salts contained in a cylindrically-shaped gelatin shell that breaks open after swallowing.
3 *Syrups:* iron salts dissolved in a concentrated solution of sugar with additions such as flavourings and stabilizing agents.

Figure 5.2 *Parenteral administration of iron*

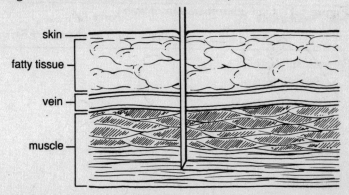

skin

fatty tissue

vein

muscle

Intramuscular injection whereby the iron preparation is injected into a muscle.

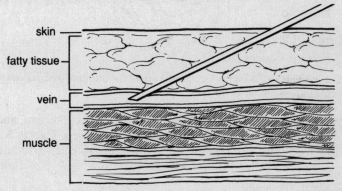

skin

fatty tissue

vein

muscle

Intravenous injection whereby the iron preparation is injected into the bloodstream.

4 *Elixirs*: iron salts dissolved in a sweetened mixture of alcohol and water; these may be highly flavoured.

Examples of a range of oral iron preparations are given in Table 5.1.

TAKING YOUR MEDICATION
● Read the label carefully and follow the instructions exactly. It is important that you keep to the prescribed dosage at the specified times.

Table 5.1 A range of oral iron preparations*

Iron Preparations	Form (✓)			
	Tablet	*Capsule*	*Syrup*	*Elixir*
Ferrous Sulphate				
Ferrous Sulphate (non-proprietary)	✓			
Feospan		✓		
Ferrograd	✓			
Ferrous Fumarate				
Fersaday	✓			
Galfer		✓		
Ferrocap		✓		
Ferrous Gluconate				
Ferrous Gluconate (non-proprietary)	✓			
Fergon	✓			
Ferrous Glycerine Sulphate				
Plesmet			✓	
Ferrocontin Continus	✓			
Ferrous Succinate				
Ferromyn				✓
Polysaccharide-Iron Complex				
Niferex	✓			✓
Niferex-50		✓		
Sodium Ironedetate				
Sytron				✓

Iron Preparations	Form (✓)			
	Tablet	Capsule	Syrup	Elixir

Compound Iron Preparations

Fefol-Vit -
    ferrous sulphate   ✓
    B vitamins
    vitamin C

Ferrograd C -
    ferrous sulphate   ✓
    vitamin C

Fesovit -
    ferrous sulphate   ✓
    B vitamins
    vitamin C

Givitol -
    ferrous fumarate   ✓
    B vitamins
    vitamin C

---

* For fuller details you might like to visit your library and peer through the latest edition of the *British National Formulary* which is a joint publication of the British Medical Association and the Royal Pharmaceutical Society of Great Britain. Alternatively, if you have lots of time why not scrutinize the 'pharmaceutical tome' called *Martindale: The Extra Pharmacopoeia*, published by the Pharmaceutical Press.

- Drink a glass of cold water, preferably iced, immediately afterwards. This will clear the palate and temporarily chill the taste buds and by so doing help to get rid of any unpleasant aftertaste.
- If you are taking a liquid preparation, that is, a syrup or elixir, that causes discolouration to your teeth, try drinking the preparation through a straw.
- Consult your doctor about any side-effects. In some

circumstances it may be necessary to prescribe a different preparation.

● Unless advised otherwise by your doctor, complete the full course of treatment. Do not finish simply because you feel better and on no account give your medication away because you think someone else might benefit.

ASK YOUR DOCTOR

Iron preparations may cause side-effects. Your doctor is the best person to ask about this as medical practitioners have up-to-date information. Adverse effects associated with oral iron therapy include:

● Gastrointestinal irritation
● Abdominal pain
● Nausea
● Vomiting
● Diarrhoea
● Constipation
● Blackened faeces
● Blackened teeth (from certain liquid preparations)

Iron by injection

If oral iron therapy is unsuccessful, it may be necessary to administer iron parenterally (see Figure 5.2, p.33). The most usual way of administering iron parentally is by means of a course of deep intramuscular injections over a period of about ten days. In certain circumstances it may be administered as a single dose by slow intravenous infusion over a period of six to eight hours.

Two solutions used for parenteral administration of iron include *iron dextran* and *iron sorbitol*. The former can be injected into muscles, and in selected cases, into veins, by means of intravenous infusion; the latter is designed for intramuscular injection only. Clearly, your medical practitioner will prescribe this form of iron therapy with considerable caution. These forms of iron are only ever prescribed in particular circumstances. They would be considered if you had any of the following:

- Difficulty in taking oral iron preparations
- Severe gastrointestinal side effects
- Continuing blood loss, possibly due to an ulcer
- Malabsorption of iron, such as after gastrectomy (surgical removal of stomach in whole or in part).

Careful consideration will be given to your medical history. For example, whether you suffer from angina, liver disease or kidney disease. As in the case of oral iron, any side-effects need to be reported to your doctor. Adverse effects associated with iron dextran include staining of the skin if there is any leakage from the needle; transient nausea; vomiting and flushing. Sometimes severe dyspnoea (feeling the need for increased breathing) occurs and, on rare occasions, severe anaphylaxis (a condition of hypersensitiveness). Iron sorbitol has been associated occasionally with severe arrhythmias (irregularity of the heart beat).

IRON AND THE NHS
Millions of pounds are spent annually on prescription medicines, and interestingly, iron preparations feature on the established list of leading prescribed items. All of this would suggest the need for iron preparations. Moreover it might be of some comfort to those of you who have been prescribed this form of treatment to know that the benefit of administering the medicine is considered in relation to the risk involved. Some iron preparations are available without a medical prescription. These over-the-counter products may be purchased in chemist shops, drug stores and health food shops. If your medical practitioner suggests this as an option, be sure to take medical advice about choice or seek the help of the pharmacist.

CHAPTER SIX
Are You Getting Your
Iron Rations?

To find out how much iron is in your diet, you will need to keep a record of everything that you eat and drink for one whole week. To do this, mark out sheets of A4 size paper as shown in the diet record diary in Table 6.1 on p.40. Be sure to fill in the record diary whenever you eat or drink anything. Do not leave this until later, as it is very easy to forget what you have eaten. Describe your foods as accurately as you can. For example, 'biscuit' would be inadequate; you need to state the type and quantity, such as 'two custard creams'.

You may feel that seven days is rather a long time for doing this exercise and might possibly be tempted to just look at a single day! A word of caution about this – food intake varies from day to day (see Tables 6.2 and 6.3, pages 41, 42) and you may have 'high' and 'low' days for iron intake. With this in mind, it is much more accurate to get an estimate of iron intake for a whole week and then to work out the average daily intake.

At the end of each day, check through the **iron counter** (Table 6.4, page 43) and record the iron content of the food portions that you have eaten. You will find that the iron counter does not give details about all foods. You can deal with this by choosing the nearest equivalent food, looking foods up in detailed tables of food composition or by obtaining information from food labels. When you have done this, add up the total iron intake for the day.

At the end of the week, simply tot up your totals of iron intake and divide by seven, as shown in Figure 6.1, page 57. The resulting figure will be an estimate of your daily intake of iron in mg. You can now compare your mean daily intake with Dietary Reference Values for intake as shown in Table 4.1.

If your iron intake is way off target and you want to increase it you will find chapters 6 and 8 ('How To Become An Iron Lady' and 'Iron Is Fun') particularly helpful. When you have read these chapters, come back to this one and use the iron counter to advantage. The useful sources of iron and rich sources of iron have been highlighted with asterisks (see key) to act as an indicator of iron content. If your intake of iron is low, it is worth considering these foods in the nutritional setting.

Table 6.1   Food record diary

Description of food portion	Iron mg
Daily Total	

N.B. You may need more than one side of A4 paper per day.

Table 6.2   High-iron day

Description of food portion	Iron mg
1 bowl All-Bran	5.4
Milk for cereal	0.1
1 glass fresh orange juice	0.2
1 cup of tea with milk	—
1 cup of coffee with milk	0.1
1 ring doughnut	0.6
3 rye crispbreads with butter	0.8
1 slice Cheddar hard cheese	0.1
1 tomato	0.3
1 apple	0.2
1 glass of water	—
1 chocolate biscuit	0.4
1 cup of tea with milk	—
Chilli con carne	7.3
Jacket potato	1.1
Side salad of lettuce and green pepper	0.5
Fresh fruit salad	0.6
1 glass red wine	1.0
Daily Total	18.7

Table 6.3   Low-iron day

Description of food portion	Iron mg
Porridge made with milk with brown sugar and double cream	1.1
1 glass fresh orange juice	0.2
1 cup of tea with milk	—
1 muffin	1.3
1 cup of coffee with milk	0.1
1 bowl vegetable soup	0.9
1 white bread roll with butter	1.2
1 orange	0.7
1 chocolate éclair/choux bun	0.4
1 cup of tea with milk	—
Fish pie	1.1
Carrots, boiled	0.3
Frozen peas, boiled	1.1
1 slice cheesecake	0.5
1 mug of coffee with milk	0.1
Daily Total	9.0

Table 6.4 The iron counter

Food portions Description	Size	Volume (ml)	Iron (mg)
BEVERAGES			
Alcoholic			
Beer e.g. draught bitter, mild, bottled stout and brown ale	1 pint	568	0.1
lager, bottled	1 pint	568	—
Cider sweet or dry*	1 pint	568	2.8
Wine, red	4 fl oz	114	1.0
rosé	4 fl oz	114	1.1
white, dry	4 fl oz	114	0.6
white, sweet	4 fl oz	114	0.7
Port	⅓ gill	47	0.2
Sherry	⅓ gill	47	0.2
Vermouth	⅓ gill	47	0.2
Spirits eg whisky	⅙ gill	24	—

Food portions Description	Size	Weight (g)	Iron (mg)
Non-alcoholic			
(Average amount for cup and mug)			
Bournvita	2 heaped teaspoons	9	0.2
Bovril	1 heaped teaspoon	5	0.7

* Iron present in *useful* amounts, providing at least 1/10 of the Estimated Average Requirement for females aged 14 to 50 years (11.4mg/day ÷ 10 = 1.14mg/day).

** *Rich* sources of iron providing at least 1/3 of the Estimated Average Requirement for females aged 14-50 years (11.4mg/day ÷ 3 = 3.8mg/day).

Food portions Description	Size	Weight (g)	Iron (mg)
Non-alcoholic drinks cont'd			
Cocoa, powder	1 level teaspoon	3	0.3
Coffee, instant	1 heaped teaspoon	2	0.1
Drinking chocolate, powder	3 heaped teaspoons	15	0.4
Ovaltine, powder	4 heaped teaspoons	15	0.3

BISCUITS
Plain

Crackers	3 crackers	21	0.4
Crispbread, rye	3 cripsbread	24	0.8
Oatcakes*	2 oatcakes	26	1.2
Water biscuits	3 biscuits	21	0.3

Sweet

Chocolate	1 biscuit	25	0.4
Digestives	2 biscuits	30	1.0
Ginger nuts	2 biscuits	20	0.8
Sandwich, eg Bourbon, custard creams	2 biscuits	25	0.4
Shortbread	2 fingers	35	0.5

BREADS
Bread from large loaf, medium sliced

Brown*	2 slices	70	1.5
White*	2 slices	75	1.2
Wholemeal*	2 slices	70	1.9
Chapatis, made without fat*	1 chapati	70	1.5

Food portions Description	Size	Weight (g)	Iron (mg)
Breads cont'd			
Naan*	1 naan	170	2.2
Pitta, made with white			
flour*	1 pitta	65	1.1
Rolls, brown bap*	1 bap	55	1.9
white bap*	1 bap	55	1.2
wholemeal bap*	1 bap	55	1.9
BREAKFAST CEREALS			
All-Bran**	1 serving	45	5.4
Bran*	2 tablespoons	12	1.5
Bran Flakes**	1 serving	45	18.0
Corn Flakes*	1 serving	25	1.7
Fruit 'n' Fibre*	1 serving	50	3.4
Grapenuts**	1 serving	90	8.6
Muesli**	1 serving	95	5.3
Porridge made with milk	1 serving	160	1.0
Shredded Wheat*	2 pieces	45	1.9
Special K**	1 serving	35	4.7
Sugar Puffs*	1 serving	50	1.1
Weetabix*	2 Weetabix	40	2.4
BUNS AND SCONES			
Buns			
Bath	1 bun	55	0.8
Chelsea*	1 bun	70	1.1
Currant	1 bun	50	1.0
Scones			
White, plain	1 scone	50	0.7
cheese	1 scone	50	0.6
fruit	1 scone	50	0.8

Food portions Description	Size	Weight (g)	Iron (mg)
Wholemeal, plain*	1 scone	50	1.2
fruit*	1 scone	50	1.2

BUTTER, MARGARINE, LOW FAT SPREAD

Average spread on 1 slice bread from large loaf or both sides of a bread roll.

Butter	medium spread	8	—
Low fat spread	medium spread	8	Trace
Margarine	medium spread	8	—

CAKES AND PASTRIES

All-Bran loaf*	1 slice	80	2.0
Battenburg cake	1 slice	55	0.6
Cheesecake	1 slice	100	0.5
Chocolate cake, with butter icing	1 slice	40	0.6
Chocolate éclair/choux bun	1 eclair	40	0.4
Croissant	1 croissant	50	1.0
Custard tart	1 individual tart	80	0.6
Danish pastry*	1 Danish pastry	100	1.3
Doughnut, ring	1 doughnut	50	0.6
Eccles cake	1 Eccles cake	60	0.7
Flapjack	1 flapjack	30	0.6
Fruit cake	1 slice	60	1.0
Fruit pie*	individual	110	1.3
Gingerbread	1 slice	65	1.0
Mince pie	1 individual pie	50	0.8
Muffin, bran*	1 muffin	70	2.3
Rock cake	1 rock cake	80	1.0
Sponge cake, jam filled	1 slice	35	0.6

Food portions Description	Size	Weight (g)	Iron (mg)
Swiss roll	1 slice	35	0.5
Vanilla slice	1 vanilla slice	75	0.6
CHEESE			
Brie	1 slice	40	0.3
Caerphilly	1 slice	40	0.3
Camembert	1 slice	40	0.1
Cheddar and low fat type Cheddar	1 slice	40	0.1
Cheshire and low fat type Cheshire	1 slice	40	0.1
Feta	1 slice	40	0.1
Leicester	1 slice	40	0.2
Sage Derby	1 slice	40	0.3
CHEESE DISHES			
Cauliflower cheese*	1 serving	310	1.9
Cheese omelette*	2 eggs	195	2.3
Cheese soufflé	1 serving	100	1.0
Macaroni cheese	1 serving	180	0.7
Pizza*	1 slice	160	1.6
Quiche Lorraine*	1 slice	90	1.1
Welsh rarebit	1 slice toast	60	0.5
CHOCOLATE			
Milk chocolate	1 bar	50	0.8
Plain chocolate*	1 bar	50	1.2
CHUTNEY AND PICKLES			
Sweet pickle	1 serving	35	0.7
Tomato chutney	1 serving	35	0.4

Food portions Description	Size	Weight (g)	Iron (mg)
CREAM			
Average in drinks and soups and on puddings.			
Double cream	1 serving	30	0.1
Single cream	1 serving	30	—
Whipping cream	1 serving	30	Trace
EGGS			
Boiled, poached and fried*1 size 2		60	1.1
EGG DISHES			
Egg and bacon pie*	1 slice	155	2.6
Omelette*	2 eggs	135	2.3
Scotch egg*	1 egg	120	2.2
Scrambled egg*	2 eggs	140	2.2
Soufflé, plain	1 serving	100	1.0
FISH			
Cod, in batter, fried	1 piece	85	0.4
Herring, fillets in oatmeal, fried*	2 fillets	110	2.1
Pilchards, in tomato sauce, canned*	1 serving	105	2.8
Plaice, fillet in crumbs, fried	1 fillet	105	0.8
Salmon, cutlet, steamed	1 cutlet	135	0.8
Salmon, red, canned*	1 serving	115	1.6
Sardines, canned in oil*	1 serving	70	2.0
Tuna, canned in oil	1 serving	95	1.0

Food portions Description	Size	Weight (g)	Iron (mg)
FISH DISHES			
Fish cakes, fried*	2 fish cakes	110	1.1
Fish curry*	1 serving	175	1.6
Fish pie*	1 serving	265	1.1
Taramasalata	1 serving	100	0.4
FRUIT			
Apple	1 apple	120	0.2
Avocado pear*	½ pear	130	1.4
Banana	1 banana	135	0.3
Cherries	12 cherries	100	0.3
Grapes, black and white	1 serving	140	0.4
Grapefruit	½ grapefruit	140	0.1
Orange	1 orange	245	0.7
Pear	1 pear	150	0.2
Pineapple	1 slice	125	0.5
Strawberries	1 serving	100	0.7
FRUIT CANNED IN SYRUP			
Fruit salad*	1 serving	130	1.3
Grapefruit	6 segments	120	0.8
Lychees*	10 lychees	150	1.1
Mandarin oranges	16 segments	115	0.5
Raspberries*	15 raspberries	90	1.5

Food portions Description	Size	Weight (g)	Iron (mg)
FRUIT, DRIED			
Apricots*	8 apricots	50	2.1
Dates	9 dates	40	0.6
Figs*	4 figs	60	2.5
Prunes	8 prunes	40	1.0
Sultanas/golden seedless raisins, raisins and currants	2 handfuls	35	0.6
MEAT			
Bacon joint, collar, lean, boiled*	1 serving	85	1.6
Bacon joint, gammon, lean, boiled*	1 serving	85	1.3
Bacon rashers, back, grilled	3 rashers	45	0.7
Bacon rashers, streaky, grilled	4 rashers	40	0.6
Beef joint, silverside, lean, boiled*	1 serving	85	2.7
Beef joint, topside, lean, roasted*	1 serving	85	2.4
Beef steak, rump, lean, grilled**	1 steak	155	5.4
Lamb joint, breast, lean, roasted*	1 serving	85	1.4
Lamb joint, leg, lean, roasted*	1 serving	85	2.3
Lamb chops, loin, grilled*	2 chops	160	2.4

Food portions Description	Size	Weight (g)	Iron (mg)
Meat cont'd			
Pork joint, leg, lean, roasted*	1 serving	85	1.1
Pork chop, loin, grilled*	1 chop	135	1.2
MEAT, CANNED			
Corned beef*	2 slices	60	1.7
Luncheon meat	2 slices	70	0.8
MEAT DISHES			
Beefburgers, fried*	2 burgers	90	2.8
Bolognese sauce*	1 serving	140	2.2
Chilli con carne**	1 serving	235	7.3
Hotpot*	1 serving	195	2.3
Meat loaf*	1 slice	100	2.7
Minced beef, stewed with onion*	1 serving	165	2.0
Moussaka*	1 serving	160	2.1
Pork pie*	1 individual pie	150	2.1
Shepherds pie*	1 serving	165	1.8
Steak and kidney pie, flaky pastry, top and bottom**	1 individual pie	165	4.1
MILK			
Average of glass, cup and mug			
Whole, semi-skimmed and skimmed	approx ⅓ pt	195	0.1

Food portions Description	Size	Weight (g)	Iron (mg)
NUTS			
Almonds	20 kernels	20	0.8
Cashew nuts*	20 kernels	40	1.5
Peanuts	32 kernels	30	0.6
Walnuts	9 halves	25	0.6
OFFAL			
Kidney, lambs, fried**	1 serving	75	9.0
Liver, lambs, fried**	1 serving	90	9.0
OFFAL DISHES			
Faggots**	2 faggots	190	15.8
Liver and onion stew**	1 serving	125	8.5
Liver pâté*	1 serving	60	2.2
PASTA			
White pasta, boiled	1 serving	150	0.8
Wholemeal pasta, boiled*	1 serving	150	2.1
Spaghetti, canned in tomato sauce	1 serving	126	0.4
POULTRY			
Chicken, meat and skin, roasted	1 serving	85	0.7
Duck, meat and skin, roasted*	1 serving	85	2.3
Turkey, meat and skin, roasted	1 serving	85	0.8

Food portions Description	Size	Weight (g)	Iron (mg)
POULTRY DISHES			
Chicken casserole*	1 serving	195	2.0
Chicken curry**	1 serving	245	4.4
Chicken pie with shortcrust pastry top and bottom*	1 slice	140	1.7
PUDDINGS			
Bakewell tart*	1 slice	90	1.4
Bread pudding*	1 serving	190	3.0
Fruit crumble	1 serving	120	0.7
Fruit salad, fresh	1 serving	185	0.6
Sponge pudding	1 serving	95	1.0
Treacle tart	1 slice	70	1.0
Trifle, dairy	1 serving	175	0.5
PULSE PRODUCTS			
Baked beans, canned*	1 serving	200	2.8
Dahl, chickpea**	1 serving	155	4.8
Hummus*	1 serving	65	1.2
Soya milk	approx ⅓ pt	195	0.8
Tofu	1 serving	60	0.7
RICE			
Brown rice, boiled	1 serving	165	0.8
White rice, boiled	1 serving	165	0.3
Pilau rice*	1 serving	190	1.1
Savoury rice	1 serving	190	1.0

Food portions Description	Size	Weight (g)	Iron (mg)
SALADS			
Bean sprouts*	1 serving	85	1.1
Celery sticks/stalks	1 serving	40	0.2
Coleslaw	1 serving	85	0.4
Cucumber, slices	1 serving	30	0.1
Lettuce	1 serving	30	0.3
Pepper, green or red/ bell	1 serving	45	0.2
Potato salad	1 serving	105	0.4
Radishes	4 radishes	50	1.0
Tomato	2 tomatoes	150	0.6
Vegetable salad, canned	1 serving	100	0.9
SAUCES			
Savoury			
Brown sauce, bottled	1 serving	9	0.3
Mayonnaise	1 serving	20	0.1
Tomato ketchup	1 serving	20	0.2
Sweet			
Custard	1 serving	75	0.1
White sauce	1 serving	75	0.2
SAUSAGES			
Beef sausages, grilled*	2 sausages	90	1.5
Pork sausages, grilled*	2 sausages	90	1.4
Sausage roll, flaky pastry	1 sausage roll	65	0.8
SAVOURY SNACKS			
Bombay mix	1 packet	100	5.1
Crisps	1 packet	30	0.6
Peanuts, roasted and salted	1 small pkt	25	0.5

Food portions Description	Size	Weight (g)	Iron (mg)
SOFT DRINKS AND FRUIT JUICES			
Grapefruit juice	1 glass	200	0.6
Lemonade	1 glass	200	—
Lucozade	1 glass	200	0.2
Orange juice, freshly squeezed	1 small glass	70	0.2
Pineapple juice, canned*	1 glass	200	1.4
SOUPS, CANNED			
Chicken, cream of	1 bowl	145	0.6
Oxtail*	1 bowl	145	1.5
Vegetable	1 bowl	145	0.9
SPREADS			
Average on bread from large loaf.			
Savoury			
Bovril	medium spread	4	0.6
Fish paste	medium spread	9	0.8
Peanut butter	medium spread	7	0.1
Sweet			
Jam, with seeds	medium spread	10	0.2
Lemon curd	medium spread	10	0.1
Marmalade	medium spread	10	0.1
SWEETS			
Fruit gums*	1 tube	30	1.3
Liquorice allsorts**	approx ¼ lb	100	8.1
Toffees*	approx ¼ lb	100	1.5

Food portions Description	Size	Weight (g)	Iron (mg)
VEGETABLES			
beans, broad, boiled	1 serving	75	0.8
French, boiled	1 serving	105	0.6
runner, boiled	1 serving	105	0.7
Broccoli, boiled	1 serving	95	1.0
Cabbage, boiled	1 serving	75	0.5
Carrots, boiled	1 serving	65	0.3
Peas, frozen, boiled*	1 serving	75	1.1
Potatoes, boiled	1 serving	150	0.5
chipped*	ave. portion	265	2.4
jacket*	1 potato	140	1.1
roast	1 serving	130	0.9
Spinach, boiled**	1 serving	130	5.2
Sweetcorn kernels, canned	1 serving	70	0.4
Tomatoes, canned*	1 serving	140	1.3
VEGETABLE DISHES			
Bubble and squeak	1 serving	145	0.6
Mixed vegetables, boiled	1 serving	75	0.5
Ratatouille	1 serving	250	1.0
Red cabbage	1 serving	105	0.5
Vegetable curry*	1 serving	220	1.8
YOGHURT			
Greek yoghurt, cow's milk	1 small carton	150	0.5
Low calorie yoghurt, assorted flavours	1 small carton	150	0.2

Figures taken from Davies, J. and Dickerson, J., 'Nutrient Content of Food Portions' (The Royal Society of Chemistry, 1991).

Figure 6.1 *To calculate mean daily intake of iron over 1 week*

Day	Iron mg/day
1	13.5
2	15.7
3	8.1
4	14.3
5	17.0
6	12.3
7	15.2
Totals 1 week	96.1mg iron

96.1 ÷ 7 = 13.7mg iron/day

CHAPTER SEVEN

How To Become An Iron Lady

You may have been advised by your doctor, dietician or other health professional to increase your intake of iron from food sources and you may well be wondering how to go about this. On the other hand, perhaps you have carried out the iron assessment exercise given in chapter 6 and come to your own conclusion that you need to up your iron intake.

Rich sources of iron

Traditionally, certain foods have earned the reputation of being rich sources of iron. Such a tribute is largely based on the amount of iron that is present in 100g of the particular foodstuff. It is relatively easy to identify these foods by turning through the pages of tables of food composition. Table 7.1 gives examples of some of the foods that have commonly been described as rich sources of iron in this context. You will note from the wide range of figures that there is little logic involved!

The whole idea of rich sources of iron needs to be interpreted very carefully and above all this needs to be put into nutritional perspective:

● Curry powder certainly gives food a distinctive flavour, but the amount used in recipes would be most unlikely to be of the order of 100g (4 oz)!

● Cocoa powder may be used to make a drink or in chocolate recipes for cakes, biscuits and pastries. Again, the quantity used would be less than 100g.

Table 7.1   Iron content of some foods*

Food (100g)	Iron (mg)
Curry powder	58.3
Cocoa powder	10.5
Liver, raw, calf	8.0
lamb	9.4
pig	21.0
Black treacle	9.2
Kidney, lamb	7.4
ox	5.7
pig	5.0
Dried fruit, figs	4.2
raisins	3.8
sultanas/golden seedless raisins	2.2
Chocolate, plain	2.4
Red wine	0.9

* Figures taken from B. Holland, A. A. Welch, I. D. Unwin, D. H. Buss, A. A. Paul, D. A. T. Southgate, *McCance and Widdowson's The Composition of Foods* (The Royal Society of Chemistry and the Ministry of Agriculture, Fisheries and Food, 5th Edn, 1991).

- Liver and kidney and offal in general are certainly high iron providers. But some people do not like offal; and what about vegetarians?
- Black treacle may be used in a range of sweet and savoury recipes, for example, Boston Baked Beans or Christmas Pudding, but perhaps we should consider the possible implications that sugar has on health.
- Dried fruit can be used in sweet and savoury dishes or just as a snack. Nibblers - watch out! You will increase your energy intakes in no time at all.

- Chocolate, delicious as it is, can be eaten as such, or used in recipes. But, if the 'sweet tooth' is not desirable or if you happen to be a migraine sufferer (migraine may be associated with chocolate), take heed.
- Red wine would need to be consumed in vast amounts which would increase energy intakes, and of course alcohol, to high levels.

At face value it would appear that foods frequently referred to as rich sources of iron may not be the best starting point if you need to increase your iron intake. Such foods need to be considered in relation to the size of food portions, frequency of consumption and last but not least in the context of a healthy diet.

Iron counting

I am sure that most of us are all too familiar with the notion of calorie counting. Similarly, it is possible to look at tables of food portions such as those given in Table 6.4 (pages 43-56) and simply identify those foods which are high iron providers without paying any attention to a healthy mixed diet. If you were merely counting iron you could end up with a bizarre and totally inadequate diet. If all you are concerned about is iron in isolation to meet the Estimated Average Requirement you might well choose to go for a diet based on any of the following for a day:

- 43 dried apricots
- 28 chocolate biscuits
- 12 rock cakes
- 12 slices treacle tart
- 7 bowls of cornflakes
- 15 beef sausages
- 2 large cans baked beans in tomato sauce
- 5 average portions of chips
- 19 packets of crisps/potato chips

- 1½ packets of liquorice allsorts

Healthy meal-planning

So, where do we go from here? How can intakes of iron possibly match up with Dietary Reference Values (Table 4.1, p.27) and at the same time produce a healthy mixed diet that is enjoyable to eat? To answer this question, it is helpful to know that iron in the diet comes from a wide range of food sources. Moreover, approximately two-thirds of the iron in the diet tends to come from plant sources. This is particularly relevant because vegetarianism, especially among young women, is on the increase. Also, the high price of meat may preclude its use in meal planning where the food budget is limited.

The secret of success is to *plan your meals around actual foods, and not around the iron content of food portions*. Use the iron counter on pages 43 to 56 as a guide in this context only. We have proved that iron-counting can result in the achievement of the Estimated Average Requirement for iron, but if a healthy mixed diet is the goal, the approach needs to be more than just iron counting. Remember the well known saying, 'We eat foods and not nutrients.'

To ensure a healthy mixture of foods, plan your meals to include foods from each of the following groups:

- Protein rich foods
- Vegetables and fruit
- Cereals, preferably unrefined

In order to recognize which foods belong to these groups, use Table 7.2 (page 62). There will of course be other foods that you may like to eat which can be very broadly classified as being fatty, sugary, salty and containing alcohol (see Table 7.3, page 64). With good health in mind, it is advisable not to over-indulge in such foods.

You need to focus on meals, rather than on foods eaten in isolation. This will ensure that a mixture of foods is eaten at a given time. If you think back to Chapter 4, you will remember that the absorption of iron from non-haem sources is

Table 7.2 Choose foods from each of these food groups

Food group	Examples
PROTEIN-RICH FOODS	
Cheese	Cheddar, feta, Edam, cottage
Eggs	hens, ducks, quails
Fish	cod, plaice, haddock
Meat	beef, lamb, pork and bacon
Milk	cow's, goat's, ewe's, soya
Nuts	peanuts, almonds, hazelnuts
Offal	liver, kidney, heart, tripe
Poultry	chicken, turkey, duck
Pulses	baked beans, tempeh, tofu, textured vegetable protein
CEREALS	
Batters	pancakes, Yorkshire pudding
Breads	wholemeal, pitta, naan
Breakfast cereals	Branflakes, Shredded Wheat, Weetabix
Crispbread and crackers	oatcakes, rye crispbread, wholewheat crackers
Pasta	wholemeal spaghetti, lasagne and pasta shapes
Rice	brown rice, Patna rice, pudding rice
FRUIT	
Berry	grapes, raspberries, strawberries
Citrus	grapefruit, oranges, tangerines
Fleshy	apples, melon, pears
Stone	apricots, cherries, nectarines

Food group	Examples
VEGETABLES	
Bulbs	leeks, onions, shallots
Flowers	broccoli, cauliflower
Fruits and seeds	courgettes, cucumber, tomatoes
Leaves	Brussels sprouts, cabbage, lettuce
Roots	carrots, parsnips, swedes
Shoots and stems	bamboo shoots, asparagus, celery
Tubers	Jerusalem artichokes, potatoes, yams

enhanced by the presence of vitamin C. So, if your meal consists of:

- Hummus (protein-rich group)
- Pitta bread (cereal group)
- Side salad (vegetable group)

the absorption of iron from all the foods in the meal will be promoted by the vitamin C present in the side salad.

Another factor that enhances the absorption of iron from non-haem sources is the sulphur-containing amino acids found in meat. With this in mind, if you were to have beef risotto as your meal:

- Beef (protein-rich group)
- Rice (cereal group)
- Vegetables (vegetable group)

the absorption of iron from the rice and vegetables would be promoted by the sulphur-containing amino acids present in the meat and also by the vitamin C in the vegetables.

Apart from iron, other nutrients appear to reap the benefit of mixing. When pulses, for example baked beans in tomato sauce, are the focal point of the meal it is important to eat cereal foods at the same time. The pulse and cereal mix will

Table 7.3 Enjoy – but caution!

Food group	Examples
FATTY	
Butter, margarine	as a spread, pastry products, cakes and pastries, biscuits
Lard	fried food
Oil	salad dressing, mayonnaise
Cream	double, whipping and single creams
SUGARY	
Sugar	sweets, jam, soft drinks
Honey	chocolate, cakes, pastries, biscuits
Black treacle	
SALTY	
Salt	foods canned in brine, salty flavourings, salted savoury snacks
ALCOHOLIC	beer, cider, sherry, port, wine, spirits, liqueurs

ensure that the quality of the protein in the meal is enhanced. So, beans on toast addicts, you are in luck!

Some years ago, the so-called high-protein diets were very much in vogue. Today, such diets are generally frowned upon – but keep this in perspective. Obviously you need to include a protein-rich food, but don't go overboard in terms of quantities and be sure to include a cereal food; if the food mixture lacks carbohydrate, more protein than usual will be used as an energy source. In nutritional circles we refer to this phenomenon as the 'protein-sparing' function of carbohydrates. In the light of this, perhaps you will view such foods as a beefburger in a bun, cheese sandwiches and fish and chips in a different light.

In addition to the optimal mixing of foods it is important to organize your pattern of eating at intervals throughout the day. Include *breakfast*, *midday meal* and *evening meal*. Breakfast is often described as the most important meal of the day and this should not be skimped on. Midday meals that are bitty are not good news and heavy evening meals are taboo, particularly if you are watching your weight. Try to arrange your meals so that your food intake is distributed relatively evenly throughout the day.

CHAPTER EIGHT

Iron Is Fun!

Getting extra iron into your diet can be fun for you, your family and friends. Healthy meal planning has been the message so far, but you will note that no single food has been identified as totally forbidden. Words of caution, yes, with particular regard to the amount eaten, but that's as far as the message goes.

Often, when people are advised to modify or change in their diet, they often feel apprehensive and concerned that the enjoyment of eating may be lost. This need not be the case. To prove to you that increasing your intake of iron can add exciting dimensions to your eating habits, ten recipes suitable for entertaining form the basis of this chapter.

Hot Punch

More than just a drink! Extra body from the dried fruits in the recipe. You can add a 'nutty' topping if you so desire.

1 tsp	orange zest, grated	1 tsp
6	cloves	6
3	cardamom seeds, crushed	3
2	cinnamon sticks, whole	2
2×(750ml) bottles	red Burgundy	2×(750ml) bottles
10 oz (285g)	dried apricots	2 cups
6 oz (170g)	seedless raisins	1 cup
1 pt (570ml)	gin	2½ cups
4 oz (115g)	caster sugar	⅔ cup
6 oz (170g)	almonds, blanched (optional)	1¼ cups

1 Secure the orange zest, cloves, cardamom seeds and cinnamon inside a piece of clean muslin.
2 Take a very large saucepan and into it pour one of the bottles of red wine. Add the spice bag, dried apricots and seedless raisins. Bring the mixture to the boil, then reduce the heat to simmering point and cook, uncovered, for 30 minutes.
3 Remove the pan from the heat and throw the spice bag away.
4 Pour in the remaining bottle of red wine and the bottle of gin and add the sugar. Stir well, put a lid on the pan and leave the mixture to stand for about 8 hours or overnight.
5 Warm the drink just before you are ready to serve it and sprinkle on the blanched almonds if desired.
6 Serve in a hot serving bowl and ladle into heat-proof drinking containers.

Note: Be sure to tell your drinking companions that the drink contains solids!

Spicy Lentil Soup

A very appetizing dish - wonderful on a really cold day. Hearty portions for about four hungry people. Great for vegetarian enthusiasts!

6 oz (170g)	red lentils	1 cup
½ tsp	ground turmeric	½ tsp
2½ pts (1.5 l)	vegetable stock	2¼ cups
1 tbs	corn oil	1 tbs
½ tsp	mustard seeds	½ tsp
2	green chillies, de-seeded and finely chopped	2
2	garlic cloves, crushed	2
1 tbs	desiccated coconut	1 tbs
6 oz (170g)	brown rice, cooked	1 cup
2 tbs	coriander leaves, freshly chopped	2 tbs

1 Pour the lentils into a large, heavy saucepan and add the turmeric and vegetable stock. Bring the mixture to boiling point, then reduce the heat to a gentle simmer. Cover the pan and cook for 30 minutes.
2 Take a small pan, pour in the oil and place over moderate heat. Add the mustard seeds, chillies and garlic. Fry until the mustard seeds have begun to pop. Caution: shield your eyes from splashes of hot oil during this process.
3 Add the desiccated coconut and continue cooking for about one minute.
4 When the lentils are cooked, add the cooked rice and the fried mixture to the large saucepan. Continue simmering for 5 more minutes.
5 Serve in a soup tureen, piping hot with a generous sprinkling of freshly chopped coriander.

Chicken Liver Bites

This recipe makes about four generous servings as a starter to a meal.

2 tbs	olive oil	2 tbs
3	garlic cloves, crushed	3, minced
1 stick	celery	1 stalk
½ lb (225g)	chicken livers, chopped	½ pound
3 tbs	Marsala	3 tbs
1 tbs	parsley, freshly chopped	1 tbs
4	anchovy fillets	4
12	capers	12
	black pepper, freshly milled	
8	slices wholemeal bread, cut into rounds 2½ ins (6cm)	8, wholewheat
4	mini-gherkins, sliced	4

1 Put the oil into a non-stick frying pan and heat gently.
2 Add the crushed garlic and finely diced celery and cook over a gentle heat for about one minute to soften the ingredients.

3 Stir in the chopped chicken livers and fry over a moderate heat for about 3 minutes.
4 Add the Marsala and freshly chopped parsley and continue cooking for one more minute.
5 Spoon the mixture into either a blender or food processor and add the anchovies, capers and black pepper.
6 Process the mixture until it is almost (but not quite) smooth.
7 Transfer the mixture onto a warm plate and cover with a saucepan lid, then position the plate over a saucepan of boiling water.
8 Make the toast, spread with the warm paste and serve garnished with the sliced gherkins.

Kidney and Mushroom Appetizers

This recipe can also be made using calf's kidneys for an extra special treat. Should be enough for about 4 people.

8	lambs kidneys	8
1 oz (30g)	butter	2 tbs
1 tbs	olive oil	1 tbs
1	shallot, finely sliced	1
2	garlic cloves, crushed	2, minced
	freshly ground pepper	
1 tsp	wholegrain mustard	1 tsp
4 tbs	Marsala	4 tbs
4 oz (115g)	button mushrooms, very finely sliced	1½ cups
1 tbs	parsley, freshly chopped	1 tbs

1 Prepare the kidneys by removing and discarding the thin membrane that surrounds them. Cut each kidney in half, lengthways. Cut out the white cores inside the kidneys. This is most easily done using sharp kitchen scissors.
2 Melt the butter in a shallow frying pan with the oil.
3 Add the shallot and garlic and fry over a gentle heat for about 5 minutes to soften them without browning.

4 Add the kidneys and cook over a moderate heat for about 3 minutes. Stir throughout.
5 Stir in the mustard, freshly ground pepper, Marsala and mushrooms. Cook for 2 minutes only.
6 Serve on hot toast, sprinkled with the chopped parsley. Eat without delay.

Choc-Chilli Chicken

Fun to make if you are feeling adventurous and have a little time on your hands. The recipe is based on Mexico's most famous dish. It is sensational in creating a party atmosphere. Traditionally served with Mexican rice and beans, guacamole sauce and tortillas.

4	chicken pieces (2 whole leg and thigh pieces, 2 whole breast and wing pieces)	4
1 small	onion, finely chopped	1
1	garlic clove, crushed	1, minced
1½ pts (850ml)	water	3¾ cups
1 tbs	corn oil	1 tbs

Chilli Sauce

4	green chillies, de-seeded and chopped	4
1 medium	onion, finely chopped	1
2	garlic cloves, crushed	2, minced
1 large	tomato, de-seeded, skinned and chopped	1
1 slice	toast, cubed	1
2 oz (55g)	blanched almonds	½ cup
1 oz (30g)	peanuts	1¾ tbs
2 oz (55g)	raisins	⅓ cup
2 tbs	sesame seeds	2 tbs
¼ tsp	ground coriander	¼ tsp
¼ tsp	ground anise	¼ tsp
1	clove	1

| ¼ in (½mm) | cinnamon stick, whole | ¼ in (½mm) |
| 2 oz (55g) | plain chocolate, cubed | ¼ cup |

1 Take a large heavy saucepan or flame-proof casserole. Add the chicken pieces, onion, garlic and the water. Bring to the boil then reduce to simmering point. Put the lid on the pan and cook for 30 minutes.
2 Drain the cooking liquid into a basin and reserve. Pat the chicken pieces dry, using absorbent paper.
3 Heat the oil in a non-stick frying pan and fry the chicken pieces over a moderate heat to brown the surface. Then set the chicken to one side. Do not clean the pan - set it aside ready to use at stage 7.

Chilli Sauce
4 Put the chillies into a food processor or blender and add the onion, garlic, tomato and toast. Process to form a paste. Transfer the mixture to a basin.
5 Put the almonds, peanuts, raisins, sesame seeds, coriander, anise, clove and cinnamon into the food processor/blender and process well.
6 Mix very thoroughly with the chilli paste.
7 Put the paste into the frying pan in which the chicken was browned and cook over a moderate heat for about 5 minutes.
8 Transfer the paste into a large flame-proof casserole or a saucepan such as the one you started with. Add about ½ pint (285ml) of the chicken stock and the chocolate.
9 Cook over a gentle heat until the chocolate has melted. Add the chicken pieces and simmer with the lid on the pan for about 30 minutes.
10 Serve hot with your selected accompaniments.

Eastern Style Lamb

This recipe is very tasty and makes an interesting main course.
Suitable accompaniments include jacket potatoes or rice and
green salad with sprigs of mint. The quantities given in the
recipe are usually sufficient for four people.

1 large	aubergine	1 large
1 tbs	salt	1 tbs
1 tbs	corn oil	1 tbs
1 large	onion, peeled and sliced	1 large
1 lb (455g)	lean lamb, cubed	1 pound
½ tsp	cinnamon	½ tsp
¼ tsp	allspice	¼ tsp
3 oz (85g)	dried dates, stoned and chopped	½ cup, pitted
3 oz (85g)	dried apricots, chopped	½ cup
3 oz (85g)	almonds, blanched	¾ cup

1 Peel and slice the aubergine. Spread the slices on a large
   plate and sprinkle with salt. Leave to stand for about 30
   minutes. Rinse very thoroughly under cold water to
   remove the salt and bitter juices.
2 Heat the oil in a heavy-based saucepan or flameproof
   casserole. Add the onion and fry over a low heat to just
   soften the onion. This should take about 5 minutes.
3 Add the meat and continue frying over a moderate heat
   for about 3 minutes.
4 Add enough water to cover the meat and onion.
   Sprinkle with the two spices, and stir thoroughly. Bring
   the mixture to boiling point, then reduce to simmering
   temperature and put the lid on the pan. Cook for 1
   hour.
5 Stir in the aubergine and dried fruit. Continue cooking
   for 30 minutes.
6 Toast the almonds under a moderately hot grill.
7 Serve sprinkled with the almonds and your chosen
   accompaniments.

All-Bran Cake

Great for afternoon tea and should keep you going in more ways than one! The cake cuts up into about 12 slices. If wrapped in foil it will keep for up to a week.

4 oz (115g)	All-Bran	1½ cups
3 oz (85g)	caster sugar	½ cup
¾ lb (340g)	mixed dried fruit	2 cups
½ pt (285ml)	milk	1¾ cups
4 oz (115g)	self-raising flour	1 cup, self-rising

1 Pour the All-Bran into a large mixing bowl.
2 Add the sugar, dried fruit and milk. Stir the mixture thoroughly; cover the bowl and leave to stand for 30 minutes.
3 Remove the cover and sift the flour into the mixture; stir well.
4 Pour the mixture into a non-stick or lightly greased and lined 2 lb (900g) loaf tin.
5 Bake in a pre-heated oven set at 350°F (180°C), gas mark 4 for approximately 1 hour.
6 Leave the cake in the tin for 15 minutes, then gently turn it on to a cooling rack.
7 When cold wrap up in aluminium foil to keep the cake really fresh.
8 Serve cut up into slices as required.

Nutty Chocolate Truffles

Chocolate has been described as an aphrodisiac! The Peruvian Indians believed that chocolate was worthy of this reputation - and Casanova claimed that he drank it instead of Champagne!

4 oz (115g)	almonds, blanched	1 cup
2 oz (55g)	icing sugar	1/3 cup
4 oz (115g)	plain chocolate, cubed	1/2 cup
1 iz (115g)	unsalted butter	2 lbs
3 tbs	cocoa powder	3 tbs

1 Toast the almonds until golden brown. Allow to cool.
2 Put the almonds, icing sugar and cubes of chocolate into a food processor and process until the mixture becomes fine in consistency.
3 Add the butter and process until the mixture is smooth.
4 Put the mixture, which by this stage should resemble a ball, onto a plate and chill in a refrigerator for 1 hour.
5 Remove the mixture from the refrigerator and shape into balls about 1 in (2½cm) in diameter.
6 Finally, lightly roll in the cocoa powder and chill before serving.

Figgy Pieces

Delicious as a final touch at the end of a meal.

½ lb (225g)	dried figs, chopped	1⅓ cups
2 oz (55g)	blanched almonds, chopped	½ cup
1 tbs	ground almonds	1 tbs

1 Mix the chopped figs and almonds together and then either pound them with a pestle and mortar or pass the mixture through a mincer.
2 Shape the mixture into a sausage - about 1 in (2½cm) in diameter.
3 Gently coat the sausage shape with the ground almonds.
4 Carefully wrap the sausage in foil and chill in a refrigerator for about 2 hours.
5 To serve, cut into slices about ½ in (12mm) thick.

Apricot Fresheners

Light and refreshing after a rich meal. Ample for four people.

4 oz (115g)	dried apricots	¾ cup
3 oz (85g)	desiccated coconut	1 cup
1 tbs	orange juice, freshly squeezed	1 tbs
2 tsp	orange zest, finely grated	2 tsp
1 oz (30g)	desiccated coconut, lightly toasted	⅓ cup

1 Soak the dried apricots in a basin with boiling water. Cover and leave for 1 hour.
2 Drain away the liquid and finely chop the fruit.
3 Put the chopped apricots, desiccated coconut, orange juice and zest into a mixing bowl.
4 Mix the ingredients together using a fork.
5 Knead the mixture lightly and shape into small balls approximately 1 in (2½cm) in diameter.
6 Roll the balls in the lightly toasted desiccated coconut.
7 Arrange on a plate and chill in a refrigerator for about 2 hours before serving.

CHAPTER NINE

Too Much Iron

Excessive amounts of iron inside the body can occur for two main reasons:
- Failure to control iron absorption from the small intestive.
- High intakes of iron from the diet or supplements.

Haemochromatosis

Failure to control iron absorption from the small intestine due to a genetic disorder called *haemochromatosis* results in a gradual build-up of iron in the body tissues. The disorder is rare and tends to manifest itself in middle age.

The accumulation of iron in the tissues causes damage. Fibrous tissue forms in many of the organs as a reactive response to the excess iron. The implications of this are serious:

- Enlarged and cirrhotic liver (cirrhosis is a term used to mean progressive fibrous tissue overgrowth in an organ).

- Bronzed pigmentation of the skin occurs as large quantities of an iron-containing pigment (haemosiderin) become deposited in the liver.

- Diabetes may develop in extreme cases due to damage to the pancreas (the pancreas has cells which produce the hormone insulin and damage can disrupt this process).

- Death can occur if the amount of iron in the body cannot be reduced.

Haemosiderosis

Iron overload as a consequence of excessively high iron intakes results in a condition called *haemosiderosis*. High intakes of iron in this respect are usually over 40mg per day, often through food contamination by cooking vessels.

Some people deliberately use iron cookware to increase their iron intakes. The iron content of half a cup of spaghetti sauce simmered in a glass (heat-proof) pan is about 3mg. If cooked in an iron pan, the amount of iron in the sauce increases to approximately 87mg. If eggs are scrambled in an iron pan for just a few minutes the iron content of the finished product can be tripled.

One common form of iron contamination results from the use of iron vessels in the preparation of alcoholic beverages. Haemosiderosis is common among the Bantu people where daily intakes of iron may be as high as 100mg. The high intakes of iron are due to the consumption of beer brewed from maize or sorghum in iron vessels.

Haemosiderosis is an iron overload characterized by excessive iron deposits in haemosiderin (the iron storage protein). It can lead to liver damage and cirrhosis and this is more likely to happen if diets are inadequate, particularly in respect of protein, and high in alcohol. Chronic alcoholics are particularly at risk. Some inexpensive wines contain up to 40mg of iron per litre. Samples of Normandy cider have been reported to contain 16mg of iron per litre.

Iron poisoning

Iron poisoning is second to aspirin as a cause of accidental poisoning in young children. This tends to happen when children mistakenly eat iron tablets, thinking that they are sweets. Clearly, if you are on iron medication you need to make sure that your tablets are well out of reach of children. The signs of iron intoxication show relatively quickly. Within an hour the child is nauseous, and vomiting and diarrhoea occur. Depending upon the amount of iron salts absorbed the condition can be severe and cause gastrointestinal bleeding and other tissue damage which is often fatal.

Iron poisoning is rare in adults. Only a few cases have been reported in the literature.

If you are on medicinal iron, keep to the prescribed dosage as previously stated in Chapter 5.

Iron overload and infection

Iron overload is associated with infections due to the fact that bacteria thrive on iron-rich blood. Bacteria require adequate quantities of iron for their replication. The following examples illustrate this point:

● Administration of iron to children with protein calorie malnutrition before immune mechanisms had been restored, such as seen in the Third World, has been reported to increase fatalities from overwhelming bacterial sepsis.

● Iron therapy for iron-deficiency anaemia has resulted in exacerbation of malaria in people living in Nigeria and Somalia.

● Parasitism increased from 5 per cent to 50 per cent in starved Sahelian drought victims when iron concentrations rose rapidly after a few days of re-feeding.

PRACTICAL TIPS
1 Avoid the regular use of iron cooking vessels.
2 Eat a healthy diet with adequate amounts of protein.
3 Be cautious about the quantity of wine that you drink, particularly some of the cheaper varieties.
4 If you are taking iron supplements, keep them away from children and follow the prescribed dosage.

CHAPTER TEN

Megaloblastic Anaemia

Anaemia may develop as a result of a deficiency in nutrients other than iron. Admittedly iron-deficiency is the most common cause for the disorder, but lack of *vitamin B12* and *folate* can also lead to a particular kind of anaemia. Both vitamin B12 and folate are needed for the normal production and maturation of red blood cells in the bone marrow. Lack of either of these vitamins seriously interferes with the production of red blood cells. An excess of abnormal cells called *megaloblasts* appear in the bone marrow and these give rise to enlarged and deformed red blood cells called *macrocytes*. The underlying problem is at the level of deoxyribonucleic acid (DNA) synthesis. Both folate and vitamin B12 are essential for the orderly production of this in all tissue cells. This form of anaemia may also be associated with a reduction in the number of white blood cells and platelets.

What causes megaloblastic anaemia?

VITAMIN B12 DEFICIENCY
The primary causes of vitamin B12 deficiency relate to malabsorption or decreased availability in the gastrointestinal tract. Deficiency rarely results from dietary insufficiency. This only happens in very extreme situations because the vitamin is abundant in most diets. There is a low requirement by the tissues and the body has a reserve which may last for approximately two years.

Vitamin B12 is found naturally in foods of animal origin;

including meat, poultry, fish, eggs and dairy products. Plant foods contain none at all unless they become contaminated by bacteria or algae. Strict vegetarians, known as total vegetarians or vegans, are potentially at risk of developing vitamin B12 deficiency since their diet is based on plant foods. In practice, thanks to the very sound nutritional advice proferred by both the Vegetarian and Vegan Societies, this rarely happens.

For 'normal' absorption of vitamin B12, which takes place in the ileum (part of the small intestine), the vitamin needs to become bound to a factor found in saliva, called *haptocorrin* and then to another factor called *intrinsic factor* which is produced by cells found in the lining of the stomach. The most common cause for vitamin B12 deficiency is due to a failure of intrinsic factor secretion. The megaloblastic anaemia formed in this way is known as *pernicious anaemia*. The inability to produce intrinsic factor is usually because of an autoimmune disorder, in which antibodies are produced that block the production of intrinsic factor. Pernicious anaemia tends to run in families, to start in middle age, and to affect women more than men.

Impaired absorption of vitamin B12 is an inevitable consequence of total gastrectomy, whereby the whole of the stomach is removed. Poor absorption may also be a feature of coeliac disease and Crohn's disease (an inflammatory lesion of the intestines of unknown cause). One very interesting reason for poor absorption of vitamin B12 is the presence of the tapeworm *Diphyllobothrium latum* in the gut. The tapeworm absorbs the vitamin, so infection with the worm may lead to megaloblastic anaemia. The worm is widespread in fish, but is fortunately not common in humans. In Finland about 2 per cent of adults carry it but only a small proportion of carriers develop megaloblastic anaemia.

FOLATE DEFICIENCY

In contrast to vitamin B12 deficiency, folate deficiency is usually due to dietary inadequacy. Body stores only last for about four months. Folate is widely distributed and almost all foods contain a variable amount. If the intake of folate is lacking, deficiency develops relatively quickly in comparison with B12 deficiency, due to the fact that a constant supply of the nutrient is needed.

Deficiency of folate is most common in the poor and the elderly living on inadequate diets. Elderly people living on their own are at particular risk. About 8 per cent of people over the age of 65 in Britain have low levels of folate in their blood. Elderly people with psychiatric disturbances and requiring admission to old people's homes have been found to have folate deficiency. Old people may have low intakes for a variety of reasons including poverty, lack of interest in food and immobility. Losses in cooking, for example, the over-cooking of green vegetables, will destroy folate. Ill-fitting dentures or the desire for well-cooked green vegetables may also be a contributory factor to folate deficiency in this age group.

The incidence of folate deficiency parallels the prevalence of malnutrition in the world and is especially common in tropical areas where the diet is compromised by poverty. In such circumstances, infants, young children and pregnant women are particularly affected. The need for folate for growth and red cell proliferation in these people is increased and so it is hardly surprising that deficiency manifests itself in these unfortunate circumstances.

Folate deficiency has been associated with excessive alcohol consumption. It has been suggested that public health action in controlling alcohol abuse could directly affect the prevalence of folate deficiency. Drinking too much alcohol can lead to folate deficiency through mechanisms thought to be related to metabolism (the chemical processes participating in and essential for the phenomena of life) and storage in the liver.

The administration of certain drugs can impair the intestinal absorption of folate. Some anticonvulsant drugs come into this category. However, the actual mechanism by which such medication leads to folate deficiency is unclear.

Folate deficiency can also develop as a consequence of certain disease states that interfere with the absorption of the vitamin from the small intestine. Disorders such as Crohn's disease and coelic disease, or removal of part of the small intestine (possibly due to the growth of a tumour) will inevitably have implications for the absorption of folate.

A mild deficiency of folate is believed to be widespread in Britain during pregnancy. Folate is required by rapidly dividing cells, as in the fetus. As well as this the increased needs for folate during pregnancy are necessary for the increase in maternal blood volume, growth of the uterus and placenta. Folate deficiency may not only result in megaloblastic anaemia in the mother, but also the birth of a small, premature infant with a reduced store of folate. One very topical and interesting area is the effect of high doses of folate in reducing neural tube defects such as spina bifida. It has been suggested that folate supplements may reduce the incidence of neural tube defects when given in high doses at the time of conception.

Symptoms of megaloblastic anaemia

If you have mild megaloblastic anaemia you may have no symptoms at all. On the other hand, you may experience some or all of the following: tiredness, headaches, a sore mouth and tongue, weight loss and jaundice (a syndrome characterized by an excess of bile pigment in the blood). If you have severe megaloblastic anaemia you may also experience breathlessness and chest pain. Further symptoms may occur such as loss of balance and tingling in the feet as a result of damage of the nervous system arising from the nutritional deficiency.

Diagnosis of megaloblastic anaemia

After looking at the variety of causes for this form of anaemia, you could take stock of any possible factors that might have a bearing on the diagnosis. This will be very helpful to your doctor when a full account of your medical history is taken. For example, if you have become a total vegetarian and failed to take positive steps to prevent vitamin B12 deficiency, your doctor needs to be informed. If you are a heavy drinker, you need to mention this, as alcohol can have a detrimental effect on the utilization of folate.

Diagnosis is dependent upon blood tests. If you have megaloblastic anaemia you will have a low level of haemoglobin and a preponderance of large red blood cells. You may also be found to have low blood levels of vitamin B12 or folate, or both. It is also possible that you will need to have further tests, such as a bone marrow biopsy (removal of a small sample of marrow for analysis). If you have megaloblastic anaemia, your bone marrow will have large numbers of megaloblasts (abnormal, immature red blood cells).

If pernicious anaemia is suspected you may be asked to subject yourself to a test called the *Schilling test*. This test will show if your problem stems from lack of the intrinsic factor that is necessary for the absorption of vitamin B12 from the gut.

Treatment of megaloblastic anaemia

The prescribed treatment will depend upon the cause. If the underlying cause for the anaemia is a poor diet, this can be remedied by making some adjustments to what you eat and by taking a short course of vitamin B12 injections or folate tablets.

If the problem is due to an inability to absorb vitamin B12, as in the case of pernicious anaemia, it will be necessary to have injections of the vitamin for the rest of your life.

How much vitamin B12 to aim for?

According to the Department of Health, the average requirement to prevent or cure megaloblastic anaemia, arising from dietary deficiency of vitamin B12, is less than 1.0mg per day. This figure is based on the findings of various studies. For example, Australian Seventh Day Adventist vegetarians did not have megaloblastic anaemia when their intakes were estimated to be 0.26mg per day. Swedish vegans, similarly without anaemia, had vitamin B12 intakes of 0.3 and 0.4mg a day. In the light of this, the Lower Reference Nutrient Intake for adults was set at 1mg per day. You will remember from Chapter 4 that the Estimated Average Requirement represents a notional mean requirement. To reduce the risk of megaloblastic anaemia in most people and to provide sufficient stores to face periods of zero intake, the Department of Health considered that the Reference Nutrient Intake of 1.5mg a day would be sufficient. Table 10.1 gives a summary of Dietary Reference Values for vitamin B12.

Table 10.1 Dietary Reference Values for vitamin B12 expressed as micrograms per day*

Age (years)	Lower Reference Nutrient Intake	Estimated Average Requirement	Reference Nutrient Intake
11-14 (males/females)	0.8	1.0	1.2
15-50+ (males/females)	1.0	1.25	1.5
Breast feeding	—	—	+ 0.5

Unlike the Dietary Reference Values for Iron (Table 4.1), the figures show that no distinction is made between males and females or reproductive stage in the life cycle. In accord with iron no additional increment is given for pregnancy, but in contrast an increment is given for breast feeding.

* Figures in the table come from 'Dietary Reference Values for Food Energy and Nutrients for the United Kingdom', Report of the Panel on Dietary Reference Values of the Committee on Medical Aspects of Food Policy. Department of Health (HMSO, 1991).

The DOH acknowledge that there is little information about vitamin B12 requirements during pregnancy. The view taken was that as long as the body had a store of the vitamin (remember, this should last for about 2 years) the RNI of 1.5µg a day whould be adequate. Having regard to breast feeding, an increment of 0.5µg a day was recommended to ensure an adequate supply of the vitamin for breast milk. It has been estimated that breast milk contains about 0.2 to 1.0µg of vitamin B12 per litre if it comes from a healthy, well-nourished mother.

How to ensure adequate intakes of vitamin B12

For the majority of you, this won't be a problem. Assuming a mixed diet including meat, poultry, fish, eggs and dairy products, intakes of vitamin B12 should be more than adequate. Trends in food consumption indicate that populations with a high content of animal protein in the diet

Table 10.2 Vitamin B$_{12}$ content of some food portions*

Description	Size	Weight (g)	Vitamin B$_{12}$ (µg)
DAIRY			
Cheddar cheese	1 slice	40	0.44
whole milk	1 glass ⅓ pt	195	0.78
EGGS			
boiled	1 size 2	60	0.66
scrambled	2 eggs	140	2.94
FISH			
fried fish fingers	4 fish fingers	100	2.00
sardines, canned in oil (drained)	1 serving	70	19.60
tuna, canned in oil (drained)	1 serving	95	4.56
MEAT			
beef-roast, lean, topside	1 serving	85	1.70
grilled, lean, rumpsteak	1 steak	155	3.10
OFFAL			
faggots	2 faggots	190	9.50
fried lambs kidney	1 serving	75	59.25
fried lambs liver	1 serving	90	72.90
liver sausage	4 slices	35	2.80
POULTRY			
roast, duck meat	1 serving	85	2.55
roast, pheasant meat	1 serving	85	2.12

* Size of food portions taken from Nutrient Content of Food Portions, J. Davies and J. Dickerson (Royal Society of Chemistry, 1991).

Vitamin B$_{12}$ figures derived from B. Holland, A. A. Welch, J. D. Irwin, D. H. Buss, A. A. Paul, D. A. T. Southgate, *McCance & Widdowson's The Composition of Foods* (The Royal Society of Chemistry and the Ministry of Agriculture, Fisheries and Food, 5th Edn, 1991).

(the so-called high-cost diets) have intakes ranging from 4.0 to 85µg of vitamin B12 per day. A mixed diet supplies a variable amount, usually from 1.0 to 8.0µg a day. A vegan diet (without very careful planning) will provide less than 1.0µg a day.

Table 10.2 shows that foods of animal origin can make a significant contribution to dietary intakes of vitamin B12. Clearly, those of you on mixed diets should not have a problem. However, if you are moving away from eating foods of animal origin or have already become vegan you need to choose foods that have either naturally become contaminated with vitamin B12 as a consequence of microbial growth. Alternatively, go for those foods which have added vitamin B12. Table 10.3 gives a list of foods that come into either of these two categories.

MISO
Miso – pronounced 'mee-so' – originated in China about 2,500 years ago, and it has been developed by the Japanese. It comes in the form of a paste and is similar to peanut butter in texture. It can be used as a seasoning and as a spread. Miso is made from soya beans which are carefully selected. The beans are then soaked, steamed, cooled and blended with salt and a fermentation starter called 'koji'. The starter is prepared by growing *aspergillus oryzae* on rice which has been soaked and steamed. The fermentation time varies: for a light variety, miso, one week may suffice. Darker varieties can take up to two years. Miso can be made at home as well as on a commercial scale.

TEMPEH
Tempeh – pronounced 'tempay' – has been eaten for centuries in South-east Asia. It comes in the form of small slabs. It has great versatility in food preparation: for example, it can be

**Table 10.3   Some sources of vitamin B$_{12}$ suitable for strict
vegetarians (vegans)**

Food	Vitamin B$_{12}$	(µg)/100g of food
FERMENTED FOODS		
miso, fermented bean paste*	0.2	
tempeh, fermented soya bean cake*	0.1	may be as high as 1.6µg with bacterial contamination
MARGARINES		
pure vegetable (Mathews)	5.0	
sunflower (Suma)	5.0	
vegetable/sunflower (Hawthorn Vale)	5.0	
SEA VEGETABLES		
kombu, dried, raw*	2.8	
laverbread	1.6	
nori, dried, raw*	27.5	ranges from 13 to 47µg
wakame, dried, raw*	2.5	
SOYA MILK		
ready to use (Plamil)	1.6	
Textured vegetable protein and vegetable protein mixes, dried	1.4–8.0	
Vegetable stock cube (Vecon)	13.34	

Food	Vitamin B_{12} (μg)/100g of food
Yeast extracts (Community, Ethos, Tastex)	50.0

* Figures derived from B. Holland, I. D. Unwin and D. H. Buss, *Vegetables, Herbs and Spices. The Fifth Supplement to McCance & Widdowson's The Composition of Foods* (Royal Society of Chemistry, 5th Edn, 1991).

All remaining figures courtesy of the Research Section of The Vegetarian Society.

fried, made into burgers and cut into strips to use in flans. Tempeh is made from soya beans which have been split and hulled. The hulled beans are boiled, cooled and blended with vinegar and a fermentation starter called *rhizopus oligosporus*. The beans are packed into containers and incubated at between 29°C and 35°C for about 26 to 30 hours, after which time the tempeh should have a white fluffy layer, concealing the beans which are held together as a solid cake. Tempeh is available from health food shops and can also be made at home using a 'tempeh kit'; this is comparable to making yogurt at home.

TEXTURED VEGETABLE PROTEIN
Textured vegetable protein, commonly described as TVP, is a well-established meat analogue. It is a versatile food, sold in dried form. Textured vegetable protein is made from soya beans. The beans are made into a flour which is then made into meat substitutes by processes of either spinning or extrusion. Various ingredients may be added: for example, flavourings and colourings. Textured vegetable protein comes in two main forms, cubes and mince.

SEA VEGETABLES
The culinary delights of seaweed, more popularly known as sea vegetables, have been experienced since prehistoric times. In Japan, sea vegetables have been a staple item of diet for thousands of years. Table 10.4 highlights some of the features of the dried sea vegetables given in Table 10.3.

Table 10.4 Dried sea vegetables

Type	Characteristics	Uses
BROWN		
Kombu	Dark strips, shredded or powdered. Rich in monosodium glutamate, and enhances flavours	Used to make stock for soups and broths, and as a vegetable.
Wakame	Delicate green leaf, with a mild flavour.	Used in soups, salads and goes well with other vegetables.
RED		
Nori	Dried sheets 18cm square, brittle, shiny with green translucency, mild flavour. Available toasted (sushi nori) and toasted and shredded (kizami nori).	Sheets used as edible wrapping in dishes such as nori-wrapped rice balls. Used in soups.

VITAMIN B12 SUPPLEMENTS

Some vegans opt for supplements to ensure enough vitamin B12. Mexican spirulina tablets are quite popular in this respect.

How much folate to aim for

Intakes of 50 to 100μg of folate a day have been found to cure naturally-occurring megaloblastic anaemia arising from folate deficiency. In an experimental situation when folate deficiency was induced by a low folate diet of less than 5μg of folate per day, the deficiency symptoms were reversed by an intake of 50 μg a day. It is perhaps not surprising therefore that the Department of Health has set the Lower

Reference Nutrient Intake for folate at 100 µg per day. The Estimated Average Requirement, the notional mean requirement, is 150 µg per day. The intakes of folate in Britain are about 300 µg per day by men, and 209 µg per day by women, and the DOH have set the Reference Nutrient Intake at 200 µg a day.

Table 10.5 Dietary Reference Values for folate expressed as micrograms per day*

Age (years)	Lower Reference Nutrient Intake	Estimated Average Requirement	Reference Nutrient Intake
11-50+ (males/females)	100	150	200
Pregnancy	—	—	+ 100
Breast feeding	—	—	+ 60

An increment is allowed for both pregnancy and breast feeding.

* Figures in the table come from 'Dietary Reference Values for Food Energy and Nutrients for the United Kingdom', Report of the Panel on Dietary Reference Values of the Committee on Medical Aspects of Food Policy, Department of Health (HMSO, 1991).

Table 10.5 shows that an increment of folate is desirable during pregnancy and breast feeding. Additional folate is needed during pregnancy to maintain blood folate levels at or above those of non-pregnant women. Interestingly, the Medical Research Council is investigating the possible link between folate supplementation preconceptually and a reduction in neural-tube defects. Additional folate is needed to meet the demands of breast feeding. The amount of folate in breast milk is about 40 µg a day and needs to be replaced.

How to ensure adequate intakes of folate

Foods usually quoted as being rich in folate include green leafy vegetables, liver and yeast extract. However, to put this into perspective we need to come back to the food portion debate.

How frequently are green leafy vegetables, liver and yeast extract eaten, and in what quantities? Yeast extract, for example, contains 1,010 μg of folate per 100 grams. In practice, a typical portion is only about 4 grams. As mentioned earlier with reference to iron, not everyone chooses to eat offal. Further to this, we have already established that folate is susceptible to losses in cooking, so figures quoted for raw foods are unrealistic if the foods are usually cooked! Table 10.6 has deliberately been included with the view of giving a more realistic insight into the distribution of folate in a range of food portions.

Table 10.6 Folate content of some food portions*

Description	Size	Weight (g)	Folate (μg)
CEREALS			
wholemeal/wholewheat bread, from large loaf, medium sliced	2 slices	70	27
cornflakes	1 serving	25	62
CHEESE			
Cheddar	1 slice	40	41
Stilton	1 slice	40	18
EGGS			
omelette	2 eggs	135	40
Scotch egg	1 egg	120	50
OFFAL			
fried lamb's liver	1 serving	90	216
liver pâté	1 serving	60	53
PULSES			
boiled blackeye beans	1 serving	105	220
boiled chick peas	1 serving	105	57

Description	Size	Weight (g)	Folate (µg)
SAVOURY SPREADS as on bread from large loaf			
Bovril	1 med. spread	4	42
Marmite	1 med. spread	4	40
VEGETABLES			
boiled broccoli	1 serving	95	61
boiled Brussels sprouts	1 serving	115	126
boiled spinach	1 serving	130	117

* Size of food portions taken from Davies, J. and Dickerson, J., 'Nutrient Content of Food Portions' (Royal Society of Chemistry, 1991).

Folate figures derived from B. Holland, A. A. Welch, I. D. Unwin, D. H. Buss, A. A. Paul and D. A. T. Southgate, *McCance and Widdowson's The Composition of Foods*, (Royal Society of Chemistry, 1991).

As with iron, the story does not simply end with the quantity of folate in a food portion. The biological availability of folates is variable being generally less well utilized from plants. Factors having an influence on the availability are not well understood but it is believed that iron and vitamin C status are important.

The message is loud and clear: go for a healthy mixed diet. Look back at the meal planning scheme on page 62 and put this into practice.

CHAPTER ELEVEN

Aplastic Anaemia

Up until now we have focused upon different types of nutritional anaemia resulting from a defective production of red blood cells by the bone marrow. We have heard about the small pale red cells typical of iron-deficiency anaemia and the enlarged and deformed red cells associated with deficiencies of vitamin B12 and folate.

Another form of anaemia can occur if the bone marrow fails to produce the stem cells which are the cells in the bone marrow that give rise to the red blood cells (Figure 1.2, page 6). This type of anaemia is called aplastic anaemia. Failed formation and division of stem cells in the bone marrow causes a marked reduction in the red blood cells and other blood cells (white cells and platelets).

What causes aplastic anaemia?

Interference with the bone marrow's cell producing capacity can arise for different reasons: radiotherapy and anti-cancer drugs used in the treatment of cancer, and other drugs and certain types of viral infection. In these circumstances the bone marrow usually recovers once the cause is removed and normal production of cells resumes.

A more persistent aplastic anaemia can occur in association with long-term exposure to insecticides and benzine fumes (a constituent of petrol). Moderate to high doses of nuclear radiation from nuclear explosions or radioactive fallout are known to be a cause of this type of anaemia. About 50 per cent of these cases involve an auto immune process (a reaction of the individual's immune system against the organs or tissue of their body).

In some people, aplastic anaemia develops and no cause can be identified. The condition develops for no known reason. In this instance it is described as *primary* or *idiopathic aplastic anaemia*. This condition is most common around the age of 30 years but it can occur at any age.

Symptoms of aplastic anaemia

If you have aplastic anaemia, you are likely to have symptoms typical of anaemia as described in Chapter 1. Obviously related to the reduced oxygen-carrying capacity of the blood due to the reduced number of red blood cells. However, you may experience other symptoms. The reduction in the number of white blood cells means that you are more susceptible to infection. The reduction in the number of blood platelets may mean that you will bruise more easily and your gums may bleed. Moreover, nose bleeds could become a real nuisance.

Diagnosis of aplastic anaemia

Having regard to the variety of possible causes of aplastic anaemia, it is very important that you not only describe your symptoms fully, but that you tell your doctor about any possible associated events. Diagnosis is based on a blood test where particular attention is given to your *blood count*. That is to say, the number of red blood cells in a given area. This test is likely to be followed by a *bone marrow biopsy*. Should this happen, a small sample of marrow is removed and examined for the presence of blood forming cells.

Treatment of aplastic anaemia

The treatment that you will be given for aplastic anaemia will depend upon why the condition developed.

● Radiotherapy, cancer drugs, 'other' drugs and infections as a cause are usually treated by blood transfusion, whereby red cells and platelets are given until the bone marrow returns to normal.

- Auto-immune related aplastic anaemia is generally treated by immune-suppression (therapy to suppress the immune system).

- In persistent aplastic anaemia it may be necessary to have a bone marrow transplant. This is only possible if you have a suitable donor. It is usual for donors to be relatives, for example, a brother or sister. This is necessary because their tissue type must match yours.

CHAPTER TWELVE

Haemolytic Anaemia

So far we have looked at anaemias that have been caused, in some way or another, by a decreased or defective production of red blood cells by the bone marrow. Another form of anaemia exists that is caused by a decreased survival of red blood cells. The red blood cells are destroyed prematurely in the blood stream by a process called *haemolysis*. The resulting anaemia is therefore described as *haemolytic anaemia*. This form of anaemia occurs if the lifespan of the red blood cells is sufficiently severe to overcome the bone marrow's reserve capacity. The bone marrow has the capacity to increase red blood cell production to about six times over normal rates.

Different types of haemolitic anaemia

Haemolytic anaemias may be classified according to their underlying cause. The cause of the problem may be inside the red cell, in which case it is usually an inherited condition. Alternatively, the cause of the problem might be outside the red cell, in which case it is usually acquired later in life.

DEFECTS INSIDE THE RED BLOOD CELL

When the red cell destruction is caused by a defect inside the cell this is due to the cell membrane (the envelope that surrounds the cell) being abnormally rigid. You will recall from Figure 1.2 (page 6) that red cells are usually soft and flexible so that they can squeeze through the smallest capillaries. The rigid cells become trapped early on in their life cycle, which in healthy cells is 120 days, in blood vessels (usually of the spleen). The red cells are then destroyed by macrophages, which are cells that ingest foreign and dead particles.

The rigidity of the red blood cells may result from any of the following:

- An inherited defect of the cell membrane.
- A defect of the haemoglobin within the cell.
- A defect of one of the cell's enzymes.

Spherocytosis is an example of an inherited defect of the cell membrane. It is a condition in which the red cells are abnormally thick and almost spherical. *Sickle cell anaemia* is due to a defect of the haemoglobin within the cell. The red cells are sickle-shaped or crescentic as a result of the abnormal haemoglobin. It is familial (characteristic of some or all of the members of a family) and is most common in people of negro origin. *Favism* is associated with a deficiency of red blood cell glucose 6-phosphate dehydrogenase (G6PD). This is brought on by eating certain kinds of bean.

DEFECTS OUTSIDE THE RED BLOOD CELL
When the red cell destruction is caused by a defect outside the cell, this is usually due to any of the following:

- Physical disruption of the cell by mechanical forces.
- Red cell destruction by antibodies produced by the immune system.
- Red cell destruction by micro-organisms.

Mechanical disruption of red blood cells may occur for several reasons - for example, when blood flows past artificial surfaces such as replacement heart valves. Antibodies directed against red cells may occur as a result of an incompatible blood transfusion, or if the immune system fails to recognize the body's own red cells. Microbial destruction of red cells occurs in malaria (a disease characterized by shivering, fever and profuse sweating).

Symptoms of haemolytic anaemia

If you have haemolytic anaemia, you will probably have symptoms typical of anaemia as described in Chapter 1. You are also likely to experience symptoms that relate specifically to the destruction of your red blood cells. The red cell destruction is so fast that the blood levels of bile pigments, which arise from red cell destruction, are excessively high. This causes jaundice to develop, whereby bile pigments are deposited in various parts of the body, such as the skin, conjunctivae of the eye and mucous membranes. The urine may also appear yellow.

Diagnosis of haemolytic anaemia

If this form of anaemia is suspected, you will be asked to provide a sample of blood. A film of blood will then be examined under a microscope. If you have haemolytic anaemia, it is likely that there are more immature red cells and these may be of a particular shape, as already noted. Diagnosis is dependent upon a careful medical history.

Treatment of haemolytic anaemia

The particular treatment will depend upon the underlying cause of the condition.

1 Inherited haemolytic anaemias may be controlled by removing the main site where the red blood cells are destroyed - the spleen.
2 Defects relating to enzymes, as in favism, may be prevented by avoiding the particular bean that causes the disorder.
3 Reducing the mechanical disruption of red blood cells relies on minimising the disruptive forces.
4 Immune or auto-immune processes may be controlled by immuno-suppressant drugs.
5 Anti-malarial drugs may be required in haemolysis caused by malaria.

If the haemolytic anaemia, irrespective of specific cause, is life-threatening it may be necessary for a blood transfusion to be given. This could be of red cells or of whole blood.

Glossary of Terms

A

Ascorbic acid The chemical name for vitamin C is ascorbic acid.

Amino acids A group of chemical compounds that form the structural units of proteins.

Aplastic anaemia A rare type of anaemia in which the red cells, white cells and platelets in the blood are all reduced in number.

B

Basal loss Refers to a fundamental or base line loss. This term may be used synonymously with 'minimal obligatory loss' (see M).

Blood count This test measures haemoglobin concentration and the numbers of red blood cells, white cells and platelets in 1 cu mm of blood. The size and shape of red and white cells is noted and the proportion of various white cells.

Blood transferrin An iron carrying protein for iron transport in the blood.

Bone marrow biopsy A procedure to obtain a sample of cells from the bone marrow or a small core of bone with marrow inside.

D

Dermal loss Applies to losses by way of the skin.

Desquamation Refers to the casting off, of the epidermis (of the skin) in shreds or scales and the peeling off of epithelial cells such as those lining the digestive tract.

E

Erythrocytes Are red blood cells, which are circular in shape and biconcave as no nucleus is present.

EAR Refers to the Estimated Average Requirement of a group of people. It represents the notional mean requirement of the group and about half will usually need more than the EAR and half less.

F

Favism This is an acute haemolytic anaemia associated with a deficiency of red blood cell glucose 6-phosphate dehydrogenase.

Ferric iron Is a form of iron in which the metal is trivalent. The body cannot absorb iron in this chemical state.

Ferritin An iron-protein complex which plays a part in absorption, transport and storage of iron.

Ferrous iron Is a form of iron in which metal is divalent. The body can absorb iron in this chemical side.

Folate Is the name commonly used to describe a group of substances derived from folic acid.

Functional iron The iron that is being used to perform specific functions in the body as opposed to the iron that is stored as storage iron (see S).

H

Haem iron Refer to the iron found in haemoglobin and myoglobin in red blood cells and muscle cells, respectively. It is readily absorbed from the digestive tract.

Haemochromatosis Is an inherited disease, also known as bronze diabetes, in which too much iron is absorbed. The excess iron gradually accumulates in the liver, pancreas, heart and other organs.

Haemoglobin Is the oxygen-carrying protein found inside the red blood cells.

Haemolysis The release of haemoglobin from the red cells, as a result of destruction of the red blood cells.

Haemolytic anaemia Is a form of anaemia caused by a decreased survival of red blood cells.

Haemosiderin An iron-protein compound, that occurs in the tissues, where it is stored until required to make new haemoglobin.

Haemosiderosis Is a general increase in iron stores in the body. It may be associated with repeated blood transfusions or more rarely as a result of excessive iron intake.

Haptocorrin A chemical substance found in saliva that combines with vitamin B12 for 'normal' absorption of the vitamin to take place.

Hydrochloric acid Is the acid found in gastric juice, that is produced in cells lining the stomach.

Hypochromic anaemia Also described as hypochromia is a condition of the blood in which the amount of haemoglobin is abnormally decreased.

I

Idiopathic aplastic anaemia A type of aplastic anaemia for which no cause can be identified.

Intrinsic factor Is a substance produced in the lining of the stomach. It is necessary for the absorption of vitamin B12, from the intestines into the blood.

Iron deficiency When the body fails to have a store of iron, the condition is called iron deficiency.

Iron dextran A solution used for the parenteral administration of iron by way of intramuscular injection and, in some cases, by injection into veins by intravenous infusion.

Iron sorbitol A solution used for the parenteral administration of iron by way of injection into a muscle.

L

LRNI Abbreviation for the Lower Reference Nutrient Intake. It represents the lowest intake which will meet the needs of some people, but intakes below this level are likely to be inadequate for most people.

M

Macrocytes Red blood cells that are enlarged.

Megaloblastic anaemia Is a type of anaemia caused by a deficiency of vitamin B12 or folate.

Megaloblasts Megaloblasts are large nucleated red cells

found in bone marrow in certain conditions, and they give rise to macroytes.

Minimum obligatory loss Refers to a fundamental or base line loss. This term may be used synonymously with 'basal loss' (see B).

Mucosal cells Are the cells making up the mucous membrane. The moist membrane lining the digestive tracts is made up of mucosal cells.

Mucosal ferritin An iron protein complex, which holds some iron in reserve in the mucosal cells.

Mucosal transferrin An iron protein complex which transfers iron to a carrier in the blood for transport, called blood transferrin.

Mycrocytic anaemia Red blood cells that are reduced in size are typical of macrocytic anaemia.

Myoglobin The oxygen-holding protein of the muscle cells.

N

Non-haem iron Is predominantly found in foods of plant origin and is not absorbed as efficiently as haem iron.

O

Oral iron Refers to iron preparations designed to be taken by mouth.

P

Parenteral iron Applies to iron preparations that are administered into a muscle or vein.

Pernicious anaemia Is a type of anaemia caused by a lack of the intrinsic factor necessary for the absorption of vitamin B12 from the digestive tract.

Primary aplastic anaemia Is another name for idiopathic aplastic anaemia (see I).

R

RNI Is the abbreviation for Reference Nutrient Intake. Intakes above the RNI will be adequate for the majority of people.

S

Schilling test A test designed to find out if pernicious anaemia is present. It will show if there is a lack of intrinsic factor, which is necessary for the absorption of iron from the gut.

Sickle cell anaemia A type of anaemia in which the red blood cells are sickle-shaped.

Spherocytosis An inherited defect of the red cell membrane, in which the cells are abnormally thick and almost spherical.

Storage iron Is the iron store which acts as reserve. It is used when the functional iron is used up.

V

Villus A small finger-like process projecting from a surface, usually that of a mucous membrane.

Vitamin B12 deficiency A deficiency state arising from lack of vitamin B12.

Further Reading

Chapter 1

1 Department of Health. *Dietary Reference Values for Food Energy and Nutrients for the United Kingdom*, Report of the Panel on Dietary Reference Values of the Committee on Medical Aspects of Food Policy, (Report on Health and Social Subjects No. 41), London, HMSO, 1991.
2 Food and Agriculture Organization, *Requirements of vitamin A, iron, folate and B12*, Report of a Joint FAO/WHO consultation (Food and Nutrition Series No. 23), Rome, FAO, 1988.
3 Gregory, J., Foster, K., Tyler, H., Wiseman, M., *Dietary and Nutritional Survey of British Adults*, London, HMSO, 1990.
4 Ministry of Agriculture, Fisheries and Food, *Household Food Consumption and Expenditure, 1989*, London, HMSO, 1990.

Chapter 2

1 Brune, M., Magnussen, B., Persson, H., Hallberg, L., 'Iron losses in sweat', *American Journal of Clinical Nutrition*, 43 (1986), 438-443.
2 Food and Agriculture Organization, *Requirements of vitamin A, iron, folate and B12*.
3 Gardner, G. W., Edgerton, V. R., Senewiratne, B., Barnard, R. J., Ohira, Y., 'Physical work capacity and metabolic stress in subjects with iron-deficiency anaemia', *American Journal of Clinical Nutrition*, 30 (1977), 910-917.
4 Green, R., Chalton, R., Seftel, H., Bothwell, T. H., Mayet,

F., Adams, B., Finch, C. A., Layrisse, M., 'Body iron excretion in man. A collaborative study', *American Journal of Medicine*, 45 (1968), 336-353.

5 Martinez-Torres, C., Cubeddu, L., Dillman, E. et al. 'Effect of exposure to low temperature on normal and iron-deficient subjects', *American Journal of Physiology*, 246 (1984), 380-383.

6 Oski, F. A., Honig, A. S., Helu, B., Howanitz, P., 'Effect of iron therapy on behaviour performance in nonanaemic, iron-deficient infants', *Pediatrics*, 71 (1983), 877-880.

7 Scrimshaw, N. S., 'Functional consequences of iron deficiency in human populations', *Journal of Nutritional Science and Vitaminology*, 30 (1984), 47-63.

8 Soemantri, A. G., Pollitt, E., Kim, I., 'Iron-deficiency anaemia and educational achievement', *American Journal of Clinical Nutrition*, 42 (1985), 1221-1228.

9 Srikantia, S. G., Bhaskaram, C., Prasad, J. S., Krishnamachari, K. A. V. R., 'Anaemia and immune response', *Lancet*, 1 (1976), 1307-1309.

Chapter 3

1 Committee on Iron Deficiency. 'Iron deficiency in the United States', *Journal of American Medical Association*, 203 (1968), 407-412.

2 Food and Agriculture Organization. *Requirements of Vitamin A, Iron, Folate and B12.*

3 Gregory, J., Foster, K., Tyler, H., Wiseman, M., *Dietary and Nutritional Survey of British Adults.*

4 Hallberg, L., Hogdahl, A-M., Nilsson, L., Rybo, G., 'Menstrual blood loss - a population study,' *Acta Obstet Gynaecol Scand*, 45 (1966), 320-251.

5 Svanberg, B., Arvidsson, B., Bjorn-Rasmussen, E., Hallberg, L., Rossander, L., Swolin, B., 'Dietary iron absorption in pregnancy - a longitudinal study with repeated measurements of non-haem iron absorption from whole diet,' *Acta Obstet Gynaecol Scandinav* 48 (suppl) (1975), 43-68.

6 Vuori, E., 'Intake of copper, iron, manganese and zinc by healthy, exclusively breast-fed infants during the first 3 months of life', *British Journal of Nutrition*, 42 (1979), 407-411.

Chapter 4
1 Department of Health. *Dietary Reference Values for Food Energy and Nutrients for the United Kingdom.*

Chapter 5
1 British Medical Association and the Royal Pharmaceutical Society of Great Britain, *British National Formulary*, Joint Formulary Committee, (Latest edition comes out twice a year.)
2 Reynolds, E. F., *Martindale the Extra Pharmacopoeia*, 29th Edn, London, The Pharmaceutical Press, 1989.

Chapter 6
1 Davies, J. and Dickerson, J., *Nutrient Content of Food Portions*, Cambridge: Royal Society of Chemistry, 1991.

Chapter 7
1 Davies, J. and Dickerson, J., *Food Facts and Figures*: A *Comprehensive Guide to Healthy Eating*, London, Faber and Faber, 1989.

Chapter 8
For recipes see Useful Addresses - Chocolate, Cereals and Meat (pp.109-10).

Chapter 9
1 Cernelc, M., Kusar, V., Jeretin, S., 'Fatal peroral iron poisoning in a young woman', *Acta Haemat* 40 (1968), 90-94.
2 Edwards, C. Q., 'Early detection of hereditary hemochromatosis,' *Ann Intern Med*, (1984), 707-708.
3 Eriksson, F., Johnsson, S. V., Mellstedt, H., Strandberg, O., Wester, P. O., 'Iron intoxication in two adult patients', *Acta Med Scand*, 196 (1984), 231-236.
4 Pierron, H., Sauzay, F., Bellon-Serre, V., Sepulchre, J., Perrimond, E., David, J. M., 'Intoxication martiala orale accidentell d'origine medicamenteuse en pediatrie', *Ann Ped*, 34: 333-335.

Chapter 10

1 Abdulla, M., Anderson, I., Asp, N-G., et al. 'Nutrient intake and health status of vegans. Chemical analysis of diets using the duplicate portion sampling technique,' *American Journal of Clinical Nutrition*, 34 (1981), 2464-2477.
2 Armstrong, B. K., Davies, R. E., Nicol, D. J., Van Merwyk, A. J., Larwood, C. J., 'Hematological vitamin B12 and folate studies on Seventh Day Adventist vegetarians', *American Journal of Clinical Nutrition*, 27 (1974), 712-718.
3 Chanarin, I., *The megaloblastic anaemias*, 2nd Edn, Oxford: Blackwell Scientific, 1979.
4 Department of Health. *Dietary Reference Values for Food Energy and Nutrients for the United Kingdom.*
5 *Food and Agriculture Organization, Requirements of Vitamin A, Iron, Folate and Vitamin B12.*

Chapters 11 and 12

1 Heath, C. W. and Evatt, B. L., 'Haematopoietic diseases', Holland, W. W., Detels, R. and Knox, G. Eds. *Oxford Textbook of Public Health*, Vol. 4, Oxford, Oxford University Press, 1985, 250-267.

Useful Addresses

Nutrition information
The British Nutrition Foundation
High Holborn House
52-54 High Holborn
London WC1V 6RQ

Chocolate recipes book list
Cadbury Limited
P.O. Box 12
Bournville
Birmingham B30 2LU

Dietary analysis service
Centre for Nutrition
South Bank University
103 Borough Road
London SE1 0AA

Coeliac disease
Coeliac Society of the United Kingdom
P.O. Box 10
High Wycombe
Bucks HP11 2HX

Colitis and Crohn's disease
National Association of Colitis and Crohn's Disease
98A London Road
St Albans
Herts AL1 1NX

Healthy eating
Health Education Authority
Hamilton House
Mabledon Place
London WC1H 9TX

Breakfast cereal recipes using fortified cereals
Kellogg Company of Great Britain Ltd
Kellogg Building
Talbot Road
Manchester M16 0PU

Meat recipes
Meat and Livestock Commission
P.O. Box 44
Winterhill House
Snowdon Drive
Milton Keynes MK6 1AX

Sickle cell anaemia
National Organization for Sickle Cell Anaemia Research
(OSCAR)
200a High Road
Wood Green
London N22 4HH

Vegan nutrition
Vegan Society Ltd
7 Battle Road
St. Leonards-on-Sea
East Sussex TN37 7AA

Vegetarian nutrition
The Vegetarian Society (UK) Ltd
Parkdale
Dunham Road
Altrincham
Cheshire WA14 4QG

Index

amino acids 11, 63, 100
aplastic anaemia 93-5, 100
ascorbic acid 11, 100

basal loss 7, 100
behaviour 18, 19-20
bile 7, 98
bioavailability, of food 11,
    26-7
birth control 24
blood count 94, 100
blood donation 24-5, 29
blood loss 15-16
blood transferrin 4, 5, 7, 100
blood transfusions 94, 99
bone marrow 4, 7, 15, 83,
    93, 96
bone marrow biopsy 83, 94,
    100
bone marrow transplant 95
breakfast cereals 8
breast feeding 23-4, 84, 90

causes 15-16, 79-82, 93-4
coeliac disease 16

daily intake, of iron 10, 57
dermal loss 7-8, 100
desquamation 7, 100
diagnosis 16-17, 82-3, 94, 98

diet, healthy 60-5
diet record dairy 38-40
dietary reference values 11,
    26-7

EAR 26, 101
erythrocytes see red blood
    cells

favism 97, 98, 101
ferric/ferrous iron 11-12, 101
ferritin 4, 101
flour, fortification 8-9
folate 79, 80-2, 89-92, 101
folate deficiency 79, 80-2
food sources 8-10, 26-7,
    58-60
  high/low iron day 41-2
  iron counter 43-56
  meal-planning 61-5
  record diary 38-40
functional iron 3, 21, 101

gastrointestinal bleeding 15,
    16
gastrointestinal tract 5, 7
gluten enteropathy 16

haem iron 11, 13, 101
haemochromatosis 76, 101

haemoglobin 2-3, 11, 14, 101
  levels, by sex 21
  measurement 16-17
haemolysis 96, 101
haemolytic anaemia 96-9,
  101
haemopoiosis 6
haemosiderin 4, 77, 101-2
haemosiderosis 77, 102
haptocorrin 80, 102
hookworm 15
hydrochloric acid 11, 102
hypochromic anaemia 17,
  102
hypothermia 20

idiopathic aplastic
  anaemia 94, 102
immune system 93-4, 95, 98
infections:
  and iron overload 78
  resistance 18, 19,94
injections *see* parenteral iron
intellectual
  performance 18-19
intra-uterine devices 24
intracellular iron-containing
  enzymes 3
intrinsic factor 80, 102
iron:
  absorption of 5, 10-13,
    15-16
  in diet 8-10, 11, 15-16, 22,
    92
    daily intake 10, 57
    high/low iron day 41-2
    iron counter 43-56
    recording 38-40
    requirements 26-30
  precipitation of 12
  replacement of 27-9

requirements 28-9
iron counter 43-56
iron counting 60-1
iron deficiency 4, 14-20, 102
iron deficiency
  anaemia 14-20, 21-5
iron dextron 36-7, 102
iron loss 7-8, 15-16, 29, 100,
  103
iron overload 78
iron poisoning 77-8
iron preparations 31-7
iron sorbitol 36-7, 102

jaundice 98

LRNI 26, 102

macrocytes 79, 102
malaria 97, 98
meal-planning 61-5
meat 9, 11
medication *see* iron
  preparations
megaloblastic anaemia 79-92,
  102
megaloblasts 79, 83, 102-3
menstruation 7, 15, 16, 21,
  22
minimum obligatory loss 7,
  103
miso 86
mucosal cells 4, 7, 103
mucosal ferritin 4, 5, 103
mucosal transferrin 4, 5, 103
muscle content 2-3
mycrocytic anaemia 17, 103
myoglobin 3, 11, 103

National Food Survey 8-9
neural tube defects 82

ALSO IN THIS SERIES:

Breast Awareness
How to detect and deal with breast lumps and other breast problems
Cath Cirket

Breast cancer is the leading cause of death of women in the prime of life. Nine out of ten cancers are discovered by women themselves, so it is crucial for all women to know how to detect any changes in breast tissue, and what they might mean. This essential guide explains:

how the breasts work and what causes disease

how breasts change with age

how to distinguish harmless 'knobbles' from suspicious lumps, swelling or thickening of breast tissue

how to carry out breast self-examination

what to do if you find a lump

conventional medical treatments

how alternative and complementary treatments can help.

This is a book for all women, whether they have tender breasts, have discovered a suspicious change and wish to make informed choices about treatment, or simply want to protect themselves and to ensure their good health.

Pain-Free Periods
Natural ways to overcome menstrual problems
Stella Weller

'It's just something women have to put up with'

'It'll be better once you get older'

'Having a baby usually helps . . .'

If you are one of the millions of women who suffer from dysmenorrhoea, or painful periods, advice like that above is not very helpful. You may feel that the only answer is to continue to grin and bear it each month.

But there are many ways you yourself can help to lessen the misery. Stella Weller provides gentle, natural treatments that can be amazingly effective. Dietary advice, yoga, exercise, herbal remedies and other techniques can be combined to provide real relief for period pain, PMS, and the other problems associated with menstruation.

Hormone Replacement Therapy
Making your own decision
Patsy Westcott

'I felt dizzy, my memory went to pot, my skin dried up and my hair started coming out. My sex life was affected, and I kept getting cystitis. I thought I was going senile.'

What can we expect of the menopause? Will it transform us from vital, energetic women into lack-lustre old crones? And how can Hormone Replacement Therapy (HRT) help? Can it fend off the misery of hot sweats, save our sex lives, and protect us against menopausal depression? Even more intriguing, will it stave off ageing and keep us young and beautiful?

Ever since it first hit the headlines back in the 1960s, HRT has attracted controversy. Few treatments have the potential to do so much good - or so much harm.

Patsy Westcott presents an objective look at the case for and against HRT, to help you take an informed decision. This book includes the latest information on:

HRT and osteoporosis ('brittle bone disease')
• HRT and emotions • HRT and breast cancer
• HRT and heart disease • different types of HRT
• self help and alternative methods of treatment • all the options open to women considering HRT today

If you are considering HRT, this book will arm you with the facts you need to make the right choice.

Menopause Without Medicine
How to cope with 'the change'
Linda Ojeda

The menopause is just one of a number of changes that you, as a woman, will go through in the course of your life. How easily you adapt to it depends on how well prepared you are, both physically and mentally.

There are many cultural misconceptions about this phase of life. Linda Ojeda explains the real issues that lie behind the common perceptions and tells you how to treat or prevent any possible problems using natural remedies.

She also helps you to:

analyse and improve your lifestyle

minimize stress

cope with hot flushes, insomnia, fatigue and osteoporosis

develop your own personal programme of
nutrition and exercise

keep yourself healthy in mind and body

Remember, the menopause need not be a difficult time. Armed with the information in this book, you can discover how 'the change' can be one for the better, and how it can be the start of a whole rich new chapter in your life.

Smear Tests
Cervical Cancer: its prevention and treatment
Dr Jane Chomet and Julian Chomet

Cervical cancer is the most easily detected and curable cancer, as long as it is diagnosed early enough.

The only way to detect it is by regular cervical smear tests. This process is painless and takes only a few minutes, yet millions of women who should be having cervical smears are not having them. Why is it so important? And what does it mean if the smear is abnormal or positive?

This book demystifies the terms used and the processes involved in keeping your cervix healthy. Using and explaining the words your doctor will use, the authors tell you what and where the cervix is, how changes can be detected, how smears are analysed, and how cervical cancer can be successfully treated.

This book is a must for every woman who wants to be in control of her own body.

Dr Chomet has been in general practice for many years, and was one of the pioneers of cervical screening. Her son Julian is an author, journalist and award-winning director of science films.

Natural Hormone Health
Drug-free ways to balance your life
Arabella Melville

Don't be a victim of your hormones!

Hormones can play havoc with your life, whatever your age. Indeed, fluctuating and imbalanced hormones can be the cause of such disruptions to your life as premenstrual syndrome, hot flushes, mood swings, period pain, cravings, osteoporosis and weight problems.

Hormone treatment of various sorts is growing, but there are alternatives to drugs and surgical intervention.

Arabella Melville, a pharmacologist and health writer, examines all these options from a holistic standpoint, explaining how a diet incorporating the right minerals, vitamins and fats, together with sensible exercise, relaxation and other natural therapies can free you completely from all hormone-related problems.

BREAST AWARENESS	0 7225 2789 6	£4.99	☐
PAIN-FREE PERIODS	0 7225 2856 6	£4.99	☐
HORMONE REPLACEMENT THERAPY	0 7225 2782 9	£4.99	☐
MENOPAUSE WITHOUT MEDICINE	0 7225 2813 2	£4.99	☐
SMEAR TESTS	0 7225 2500 1	£3.99	☐
FIBROIDS	0 7225 2801 9	£4.99	☐
CYSTITIS	0 7225 2693 8	£3.99	☐
ENDOMETRIOSIS	0 7225 2845 0	£4.99	☐
P.I.D. AND CHLAMYDIA	0 7225 2608 3	£3.99	☐
OSTEOPOROSIS	0 7225 2509 5	£3.99	☐
BLADDER PROBLEMS	0 7225 2508 7	£3.99	☐
THRUSH	0 7225 2503 6	£3.99	☐
NATURAL HORMONE HEALTH	0 7225 2815 9	£4.99	☐
PREMENSTRUAL SYNDROME	0 7225 2684 9	£4.99	☐

All these books are available from your local bookseller or can be ordered direct from the publishers.

To order direct just tick the titles you want and fill in the form below:

Name:_____

Address:_____

_____

_____ Postcode: _____

Send to: Thorsons Mail Order, Dept 3, HarperCollins*Publishers*, Westerhill Road, Bishopbriggs, Glasgow G64 2QT.
Please enclose a cheque or postal order or your authority to debit your Visa/Access account —

Credit card no: _____

Expiry date: _____

Signature:_____

— up to the value of the cover price plus:
UK & BFPO: Add £1.00 for the first book and 25p for each additional book ordered.
Overseas orders including Eire: Please add £2.95 service charge. Books will be sent by surface mail but quotes for airmail despatches will be given on request.

24 HOUR TELEPHONE ORDERING SERVICE FOR ACCESS/VISA CARDHOLDERS — TEL: 041 772 2281.